Collins

Anne Rainey.

Health & Social Care

for Ed...

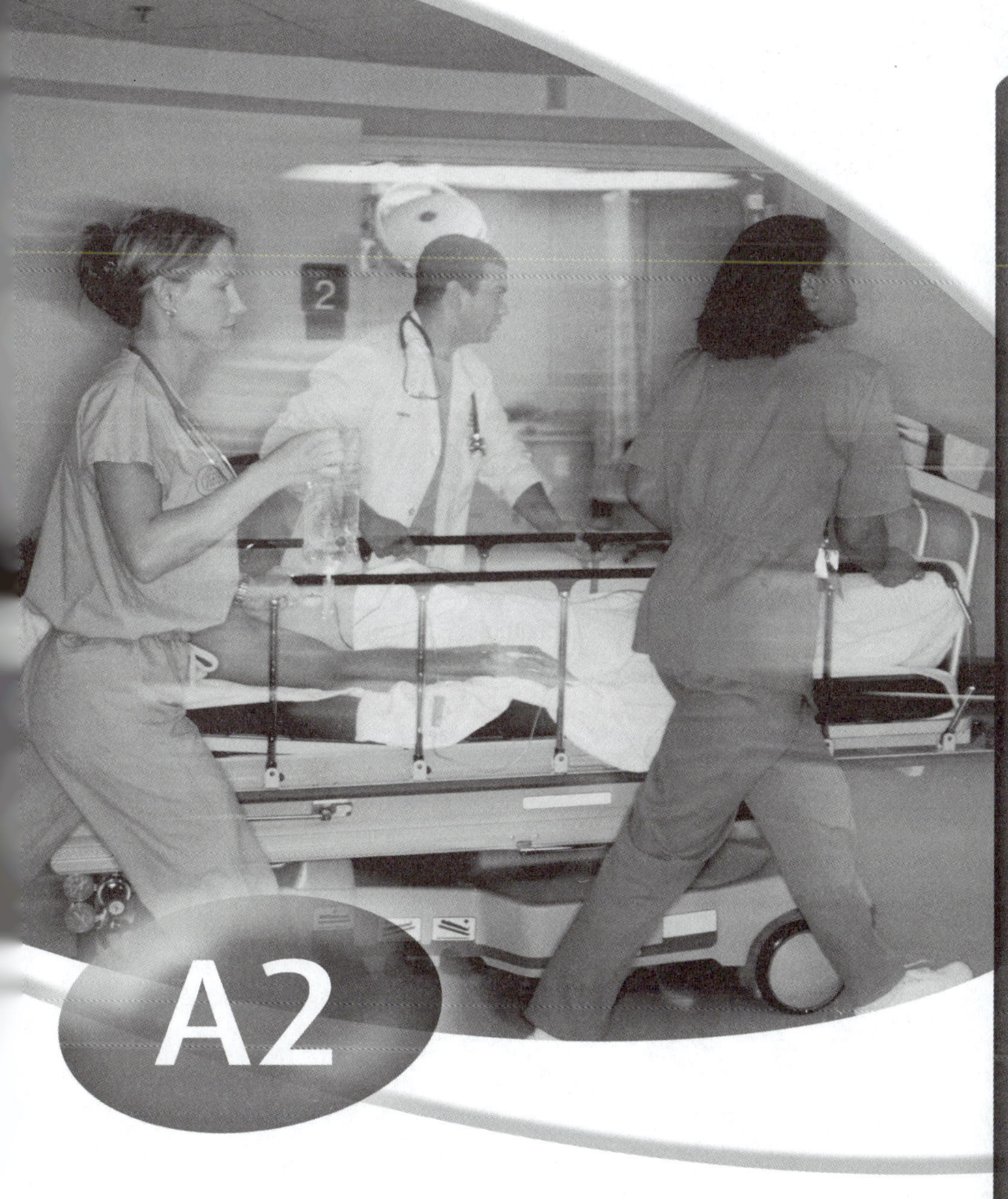

A2

RESOURCE PACK

Alison Thomson
Marilyn Billingham
Paul Stephens
Mary Crittenden

Contents

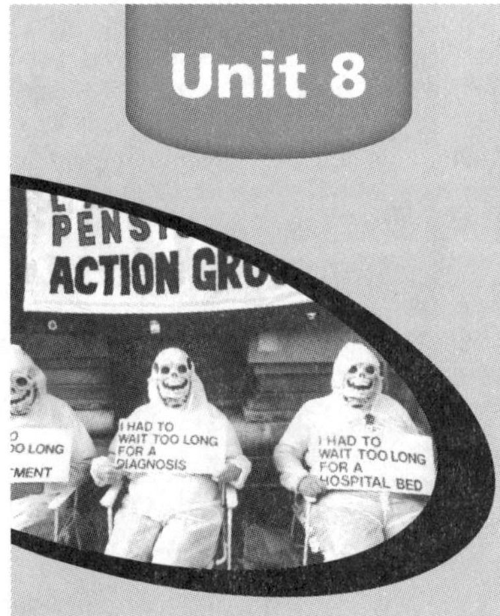

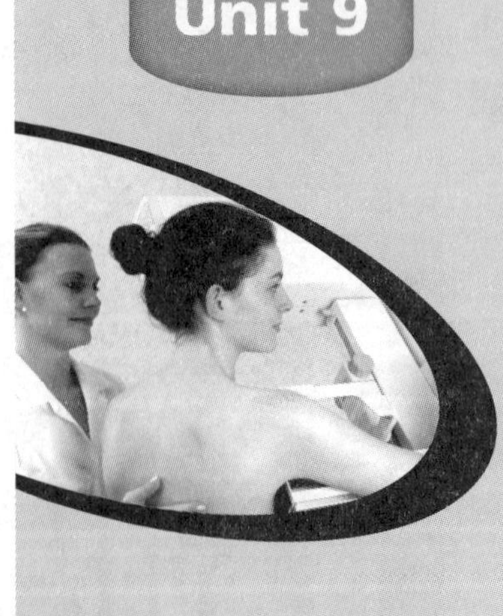

Unit 10

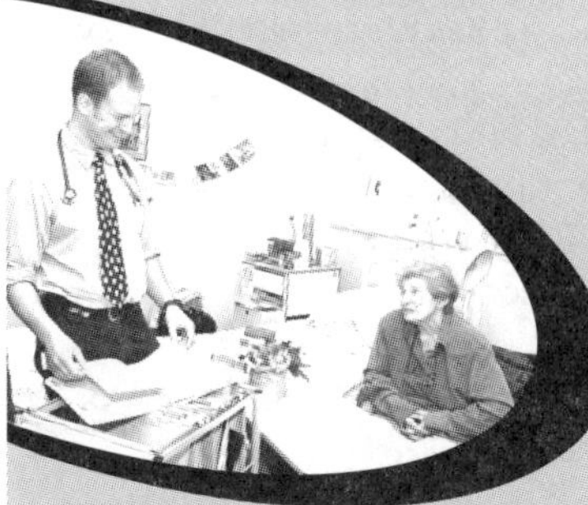

Understanding Research in Health and Social Care

Unit 11

Social Issues and Welfare Needs

Unit 12

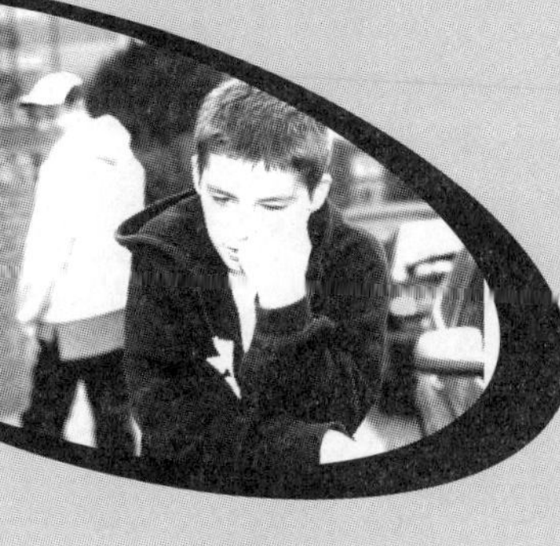

Understanding Human Behaviour

William Collins' dream of knowledge for all began with the publication of his first book in 1819. A self-educated mill worker, he not only enriched millions of lives, but also founded a flourishing publishing house. Today, staying true to this spirit, Collins books are packed with inspiration, innovation and practical expertise. They place you at the centre of a world of possibility and give you exactly what you need to explore it.

Collins. Do more.

Published by Collins
An imprint of HarperCollins*Publishers*
77–85 Fulham Palace Road
Hammersmith
London
W6 8JB

Browse the complete Collins catalogue at
www.collinseducation.com

10 9 8 7 6 5 4 3 2 1

ISBN-13 978 0 00 720044 3
ISBN-10 0 00 720044 7

British Library Cataloguing in Publication Data
A Catalogue record for this publication is available from the British Library

Commissioned and edited by Graham Bradbury

Cover Design by Blue Pig Design Limited

Cover image courtesy of Getty Images

Page design and layout by Ken Vail Graphic Design

Production by Sarah Robinson

Printed and bound by Martins the Printers, Berwick-upon-Tweed

---

This high quality material is endorsed by Edexcel and has been through a rigorous quality assurance programme to ensure that it is a suitable companion to the specification for both learners and teachers. This does not mean that its contents will be used verbatim when setting examinations nor is it to be read as being the official specification – a copy of which is available at www.edexcel.org.uk

How to use this pack

This pack is designed to complement the Collins *Health & Social Care A2 for Edexcel* textbook and support your teaching of the six A2-level units. Using this pack and textbook together will provide an excellent teaching tool and a comprehensive set of study material for the students. We believe this pack will make studying for A2 Health and Social Care an active process for the students and will enable the best grade possible.

The Collins *Health & Social Care for Edexcel* textbook mirrors the Edexcel specification. The textbook authors have subdivided each unit into eight or nine lesson-size topics that have a similar format, ensuring both ease of access to the content and a sound pedagogical approach to the delivery:

In this pack, first the rationale behind each topic is explained. Then suggested **Answers** to the *Check your understanding* questions are provided, for individual use or as the basis for discussion. **Short questions and activities** guide students through the text sequentially and help understanding and learning. Preparing the answers will also provide students with a good summary of the material, as will the **Summary worksheets** provided for each topic. Finally, **Extension activity sheets** provide opportunities for students to take their knowledge and understanding further.

USING THE CD-ROM

The **CD-ROM**, inside the front cover, contains the whole of this pack in pdf format, in a single file named H&SC_A2.pdf.

The CD-ROM can be read by Adobe® Acrobat® Reader. If your computer doesn't have Acrobat Reader software, you can download it from Adobe's website at www.adobe.com/products/acrobat/readstep2_allversions.html.

You can navigate your way around the CD-ROM, using the 'bookmarks' on the left-hand side of the screen. To go to the destination specified by a bookmark, click on the bookmark name or double-click the page icon to the left of the bookmark name.

Meeting Individual Needs is an externally tested unit and will require students to answer questions on aspects of all the different care settings: health, early years (care and education), care of older people, and individuals with specific needs. Students will be expected to demonstrate knowledge and understanding of the material in the specification. They will also be expected to apply their knowledge and understanding to unfamiliar situations. In addition, there will be opportunities for the students to demonstrate their research and analytical skills and also to make evaluations of material presented to them. Students should have an understanding of the structure and provision of care services in the United Kingdom, along with the legal framework in which care organisations and care practitioners operate. They should understand how care services are tailored to meet the needs of an individual and the role of care practitioners in providing this care and in promoting a positive care environment. They should also understand the necessity of quality assurance and how it is carried out. Many of the questions will relate to real-life case studies, and practice in answering questions relating to case studies will help students prepare well for the examination.

Unit 7

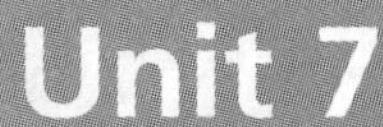

Meeting Individual Needs

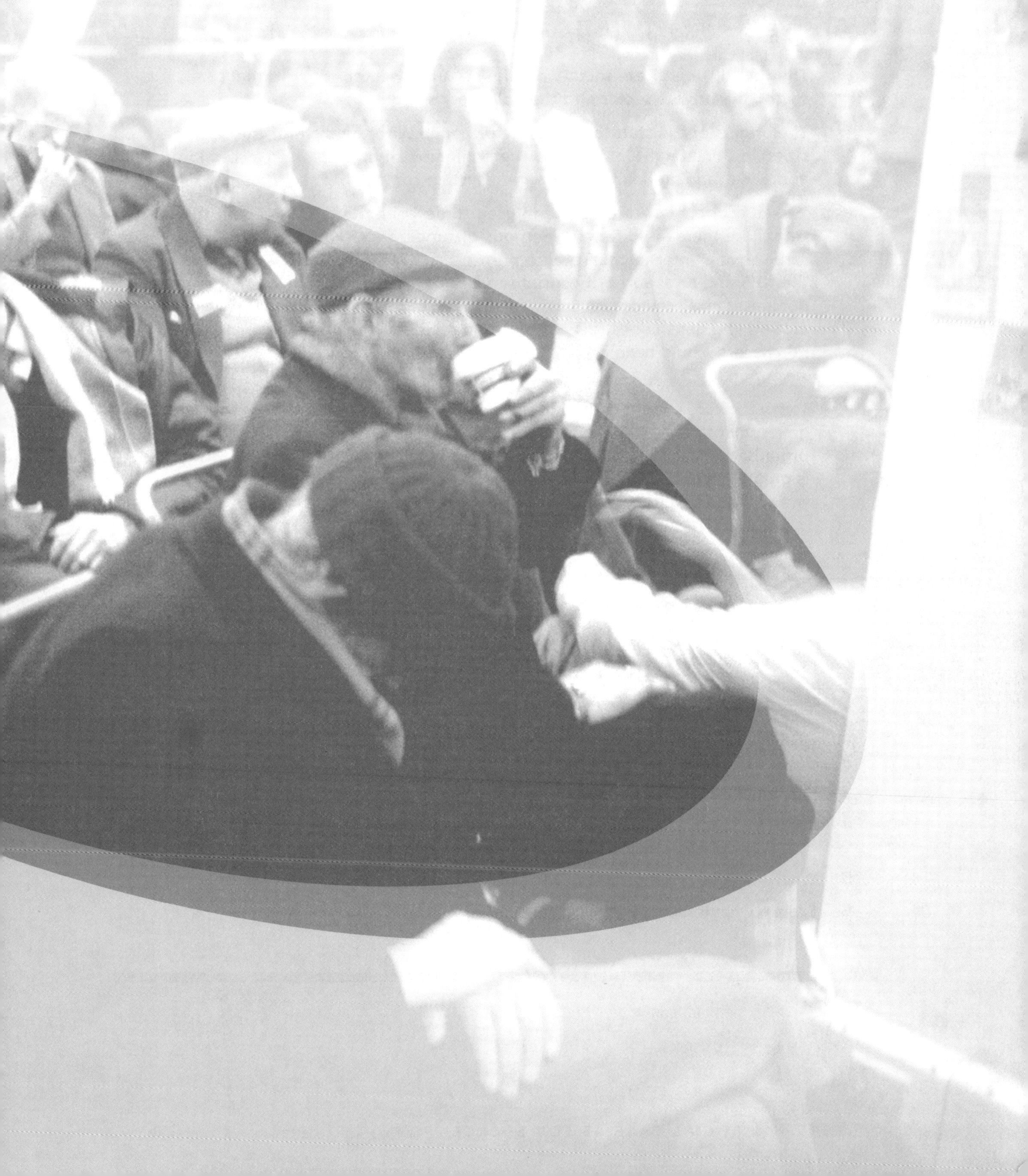

7.1 Understanding the UK care system

This topic introduces the student to the wide variety of health, social care and welfare services that are currently provided to meet individuals' needs in the UK. This may appear to be complicated for many students and they are shown ways in which the different services are grouped. Primary, secondary and tertiary services are defined and explained. The four categories of care service are explained and examples are given of each. The story of the welfare state is told, along with some of the changes that have occurred from its inception until the present day.

The case study in the *Getting you thinking* section is designed to introduce the students to some of the different types of health care services. They will see that there are different types of service depending on the ability to be able to pay. It should stimulate a discussion about the differences between health care services and social care services.

Answers to the *Check your understanding* questions on page 13 of the Collins textbook.

1 **The four different care sectors are the statutory sector, the informal care sector, the private sector and the voluntary sector.**

2 **The origins of the statutory care sector began with the birth of the 'welfare state' in the late 1940s. This was the beginning of an organised, accessible and wide-ranging health and welfare system for all citizens.**

3 **'Mixed economy of care' is a term used to describe the care system in the UK where there are different methods of funding to support each of the care sectors. 'Internal market' is a phrase that was introduced when parts of the NHS and local authority social services departments were split into purchaser and provider sections. This was to allow the purchasers to shop around and get the best deals from the providers. The idea was that purchasers would have choice, be able to cut costs, reduce inefficiency and save money.**

4 **Today the care system, although receiving most of its funding from central government, relies heavily on the private and voluntary sector care organisations and private practitioners to actually deliver its services. There is greater competition between care providers and a stronger focus on both the cost and quality of public (statutory) sector care services because of this.**

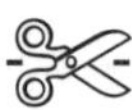

These questions guide you through the topic. If you need help to answer them, look at pages 10–13 of the Collins textbook.

7.1 short **questions** and **activities**

1 Explain the difference between primary, secondary and tertiary health care.

2 What is the main example of the statutory health care sector?

3 Give a definition of social care.

4 What are the five 'evils' that Sir William Beveridge believed had to be overcome in order to improve the health and well-being of the nation?

5 When was the 'golden era' and why was it so called?

6 Explain what is meant by 'eligibility criteria'.

summary worksheet

WHICH TYPE OR CATEGORY OF CARE?

a Health care may be primary, secondary or tertiary. Place a tick in the appropriate box against each type of care.

Example of type of care	*Primary care*	*Secondary care*	*Tertiary care*
Visiting a GP			
Having an ingrown toenail removed in the Outpatients Department			
Having a filling at a dental surgery			
Being a patient at a hospice			
Having stitches taken out by a nurse in a health practice			
Having radiotherapy treatment at a national centre for cancer			
Treatment in a residential care home for long-term depression			
Physiotherapy at a local hospital, after breaking a leg			

b There are four main categories of care service:

• statutory • private • voluntary • informal.

For each of the following examples, explain which category it belongs to:

i Social work services provided by a local authority

....

....

ii Age Concern advice and support services for older people

....

....

iii BUPA private hospital care for cosmetic surgery

....

....

THE 'WELFARE STATE'

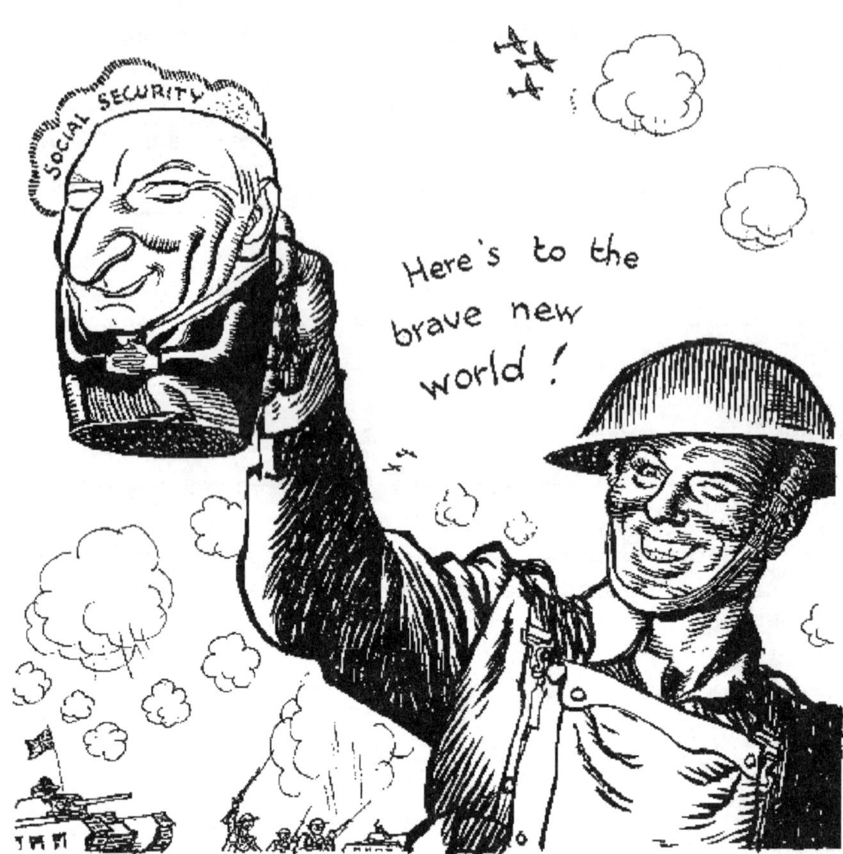

a Explain to a layperson as clearly as you can what is meant by the 'welfare state'.

b Using the information in the textbook, create a 'timeline' table summarising the main features of the 'welfare state' from its beginning until the present day.

c Using the internet and any other resources you have access to, add further information to your timeline.

d Compare your timeline with that of other members in your class.

7.2 The legal framework of care

The topic starts with the key pieces of legislation that helped form the basis of the welfare state and looks at the legislation that successive governments have introduced since then. The topic then focuses on key recent pieces of legislation that help protect the most vulnerable people in society – the Children Act (1989), the Mental Health Act (1983) and the Disability Discrimination Act (1995). There are case studies to illustrate to the students the most important aspects of these. The students are also introduced to the Human Rights Act (1998) and the NHS and Community Care Act (1990) and shown the importance of how they relate to care environments. It is important that students know the details of these acts and can show how they apply to case studies they will meet in the examination.

The pictures in the *Getting you thinking* section are powerful ones, and should help the students realise the importance of having legislation relating to the care of vulnerable people. The questions should stimulate discussion and enable students to air their views prior to learning the details about current legislation and its development.

Answers to the *Check your understanding* questions on page 19 of the Collins textbook.

1 **Examples of care legislation that seek to protect the rights of vulnerable groups of care service users are the Children Act (1989), the Mental Health Act (1983) and the Disability Discrimination Act (1995).**

2 **The NHS and Community Care Act (1990) resulted in a restructuring of the care system in the UK. It ended a long-standing state monopoly (in the form of the NHS and local authorities) on the provision of statutory health and social care services. It introduced the idea of an 'internal market'. This changed the state from being a 'provider' of services to an 'enabler' of access to statutory and non-statutory care services. This means that the role and influences of private and voluntary sector providers have increased.**

3 **Care practitioners should be aware of the provisions of the Human Rights Act (1998) as it entitles people resident in the UK to seek legal redress for infringements of their human rights by a 'public authority'. The Human Rights Act (1998) gives care services' users explicit rights that have, in the past, sometimes been ignored or denied to them by powerful care professionals. Service user groups/pressure groups and legally aware individuals now seek to enforce these rights. This must be taken into account by all care practitioners who wish to avoid litigation and compensation claims.**

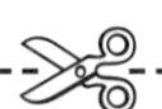

These questions guide you through the topic. If you need help to answer them, look at pages 14–19 of the Collins textbook.

7.2 short **questions** and **activities**

1. Name, and describe in your own words, the four key pieces of legislation that helped form the basis of the welfare state in Britain.
2. Describe what successive governments since 1948 have used legislation for.
3. Explain what is meant by the 'paramountcy principle' in the Children Act (1989).
4. List the different people who are affected by the Children Act (1989).
5. What percentage of mental health service users are informal (voluntary) patients? How do the legal rights of those patients compare with those of formal patients?
6. What happens when someone is 'sectioned'?
7. What four areas does the Disability Discrimination Act (1995) relate to?
8. Eight examples of clients' rights under the Human Rights Act (1998) are given in the diagram on page 18. Choose two of these and explain in your own words what they mean.

summary worksheet

WHICH ACT?

The following acts protect vulnerable people in society:

- The Children Act (1989)
- The Mental Health Act (1983)
- The Disability Discrimination Act (1995)

a Identify which of the acts each of the following descriptions relates to.

i The Act limits the length of time that a person can be detained.

ii Parents continue to have responsibility for their children even when their children are no longer living with them.

iii Contains sections that are known as the 'civil sections'.

iv Public buildings and other facilities such as road crossings and toilets must be made fully accessible for all users.

b Look at the tables on page 16 about the Mental Health Act (1983) and the Mental Health (Scotland) Act (1984) and answer the following questions:

i What is the difference between the doctors' and nurses' holding powers?

ii Give two differences between the acts relating to admissions.

WRITING CASE STUDIES

a Read the case study about Sally Hughes on page 16. Then look at the six principles of the Children Act on page 15. Rewrite the case study and include a client to which all of the principles could apply.

b Read the case study about Natalie Henry on page 17. Then read the paragraphs about sectioning on page 16. Write a case study in which someone like Natalie works with a client who is sectioned. Explain how the details you include in your case study relate to the Mental Health Act (1983).

c Read the case study about Virginia James on page 17. List the problems relating to the Disability Discrimination Act (1995) that Virginia comes across in her everyday life. Write a letter to a shop manager, similar to the one that Virginia might have written, including details of the problems she has encountered. Refer the shop manager to relevant websites.

7.3 Patterns of service provision

This topic looks at the national provision of care services in the UK. This may seem a bit bewildering to the students at first, but should become clearer as the different tiers (levels) are explained. The situation is made a little more complicated because of differences in Wales, Scotland and Northern Ireland compared to England. The different roles of central and local government are compared. Students may be able to relate more easily to the services at a local level. The importance of the internal market should be stressed in providing effective and seamless care services.

The 'newspaper headlines' should stimulate a good discussion. Students are likely to have strong opinions about cuts in services and private care. The students may have their own ideas about what is meant by central and local government before studying the topic, and they may well know about some of the health care and social care issues in their area. It would be interesting to revisit these questions after studying the topic.

Answers to the *Check your understanding* questions on page 23 of the Collins textbook.

1 **Care is organised at national, regional and local level throughout the UK.**

2 **The role of central government in the care system is to develop and plan national health and social care policies, monitor and have ultimate accountability for national care service provision, and allocate funding for care services to statutory provider organisations.**

3 **Whilst central government is responsible for major policy development and makes any fundamental decisions relating to health and social care services and the funding of care services, it is the local government who carries out the actual planning and delivery of these services locally. The local authorities are ultimately responsible to central government.**

4 **Inter-agency working and joint health and social care organisations are particularly important where client groups have complex needs that span the health and social care 'divide', and they mean that care services can become effective and seamless. This makes care provision more efficient and flexible, avoiding overlap of provision.**

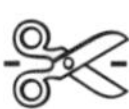

These questions guide you through the topic. If you need help to answer them, look at pages 20–23 of the Collins textbook.

7.3 short **questions** and **activities**

1 Explain why health and social care services are organised differently in England, Wales, Scotland and Northern Ireland.

2 There are six similarities given in the way that health and social care services are organised in England, Wales, Scotland and Northern Ireland. Rewrite these in your own words, as simply and clearly as you can.

3 Give one disadvantage of health care and social care operating in parallel and how this has been overcome.

4 Explain what is meant by a 'statutory' organisation.

5 Describe the difference in the local government structure between England, Wales, Scotland and Northern Ireland.

6 What is the name of the key central government department in England that coordinates the health and social care services? Who staffs this department? Who leads this department?

7 Identify three examples of recent central government care policies.

summary worksheet

ORGANISATIONAL TIERS (LEVELS) IN THE UK HEALTH SYSTEM

a Complete the table to show the different levels of care in the different parts of the UK.

	Tiers		
	National	***Regional***	***Local***
England	Parliament/Department of Health		NHS trust/GP practices
Wales	National Assembly	Regional government offices	
Scotland		Health boards	Primary care trust/ Local health care co-operative
Northern Ireland	NI Assembly/ Department of Health and Social Services	Health and social services (HSS) boards	

b Outline the role of central government in the UK.

c Outline the role of local government in the UK.

WORKING TOGETHER IN CARE

Read the case study (page 21) about Martin Jones, the community psychiatric nurse.

a Who employs Martin?

b Who are the clients in this case study?

c Describe the different ways that the clients have come to be referred to Martin.

d List the different groups of care professionals in this case study and say what skills each of these groups of workers would have.

e What is the main aim of Martin and the other workers?

f List the different ways that Martin supports (i) the clients and (ii) the other workers.

g Discuss the benefits of multi-disciplinary collaborative working.

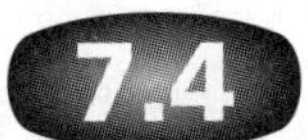 Care provision in England and Wales

This topic looks in detail at the organisation of care services in England and in Wales. Similarities and difference are highlighted, and the questions and worksheets here are designed to reinforce these. Students should pay particular attention to the way in which health services and social services are sometimes together and sometimes separate.

The picture in the *Getting you thinking* section is quite emotive. The woman is clearly unwell and is unsure where to go to for help. Students may well have fairly strong views about the woman going to an accident and emergency department, whilst others may well have fairly strong views about her being turned away. The answers to the questions there are given in the topic, but the students should be encouraged to have a go at answering them before they study the topic in detail. They may be surprised at how much they know already.

Answers to the *Check your understanding* questions on page 27 of the Collins textbook.

1 **Primary care trusts are responsible for assessing primary health care needs and commissioning primary health care services in England.**

2 **Local health boards and local authority social services departments are responsible for assessing care needs and commissioning local services in Wales.**

3 **Sources of secondary health care services in England are hospitals, and community-based practitioners.**

4 **A person with social care needs living in England could obtain appropriate support or care services through a local authority social worker or care manager.**

5 **Local authorities use a single assessment process where they simultaneously assess the health and social care needs of all adults referred to them. If appropriate, a care package will be purchased, and this could be from and delivered by statutory, private or voluntary sector social care providers. Local authorities in England are responsible for assessing and enabling access to statutory social work, social care and education services.**

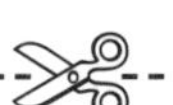

These questions guide you through the topic. If you need help to answer them, look at pages 24-27 of the Collins textbook.

7.4 short **questions** and **activities**

1. What factors have led to the care system in England being complicated and consisting of a large number of different organisations and structures?
2. What is the difference in the way in which the statutory health care services and the statutory social care services are organised in England?
3. Who runs the Department of Health?
4. The NHS and Community Care Act (1990) reorganised the statutory care sector into a 'purchaser/provider' system. What is a 'purchaser/provider' system?
5. What happened to the care system in Wales in 1999?
6. In Wales, which is more similar to the situation in England – the organisation of care or the delivery of care?
7. What does a person in England or Wales normally have to do before they can gain access to services?
8. Name three examples of specialist care that is offered through the private sector.

summary worksheet

ENGLISH AND WELSH CARE STRUCTURES

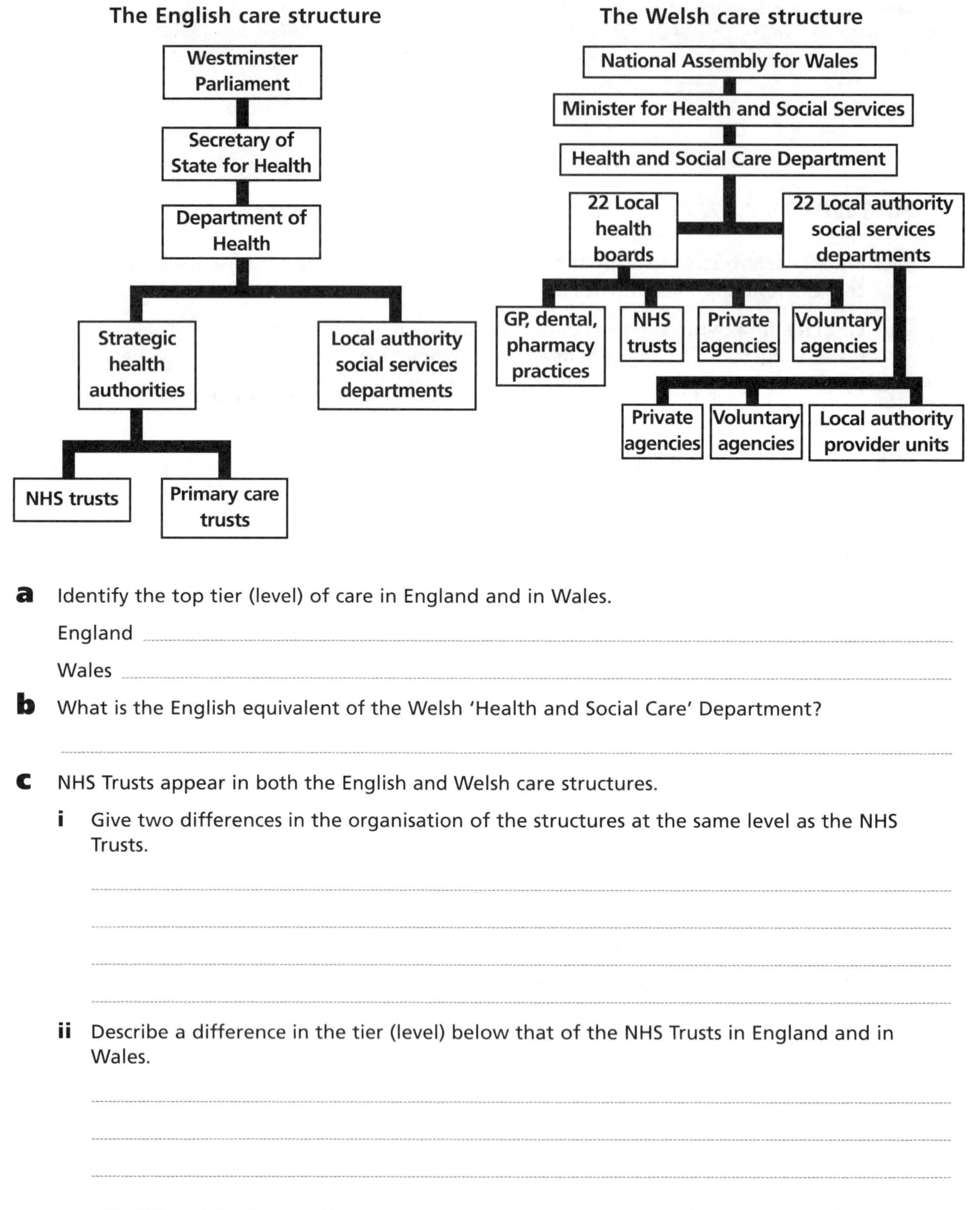

a Identify the top tier (level) of care in England and in Wales.

England ....

Wales ....

b What is the English equivalent of the Welsh 'Health and Social Care' Department?

....

c NHS Trusts appear in both the English and Welsh care structures.

i Give two differences in the organisation of the structures at the same level as the NHS Trusts.

....

ii Describe a difference in the tier (level) below that of the NHS Trusts in England and in Wales.

....

extension**activity**sheet

SORTING OUT THE DIFFERENCES IN CARE IN ENGLAND AND WALES

(You may find it helpful to work with a partner for these activities.)

Topic 4 gives detailed differences in the way that care services are organised and delivered.

a Construct a summary table that highlights the similarities and differences between how the care services are organised in England and in Wales.

b Construct another summary table that highlights the similarities and differences between the way in which care services are delivered in England and in Wales.

c Identify one particularly good feature of the care system in one country that does not occur in the other. Give a reason for your choice of answer.

Care provision in Northern Ireland and Scotland

This topic deals with the way in which care services are organised in Northern Ireland and in Scotland. Northern Ireland is particularly complicated as there are proposed changes about to happen there, transferring the power from the Westminster Parliament to the Northern Ireland Assembly. Power has already been devolved from the Westminster Parliament to the Scottish Parliament. This may all seem quite complicated at first to students, but the key points are well illustrated and the questions, activities and worksheets are designed to lead the student through the material.

Students are invited to consider data on lung cancer that relates to the individual countries within the UK. This should get them thinking about regional differences in health and thus in health care.

Answers to the *Check your understanding* questions on page 31 of the Collins textbook.

1 **Fundamental policy decisions in Northern Ireland are currently made by Westminster, but may well be made by the Northern Ireland Assembly in the future. In Scotland, fundamental policy decisions are now made by the Scottish Parliament.**

2 **In Northern Ireland the internal market promoting competition between statutory and other care providers is monitored by the health and social services board for an area. Because of the integrated health and social services the trusts are based solely on the delivery of community health and social services. Fundholding GPs and health and social services boards are able to purchase care services from the 'mixed economy' of care providers that exist.**

3 **In Scotland, social care services are provided through local authorities' social services departments, private agencies and voluntary organisations. The purchasing section of the local authority assesses need, and then purchases care from private agencies, voluntary agencies or its own provider unit.**

4 **An example of a similarity between the care systems in Scotland and England is that they are both run by government departments within the country, whereas in Northern Ireland, at present, the statutory care is run by Westminster. Scotland, England and Wales all have separate health and social care organisations whereas these are integrated in Northern Ireland. In Scotland local authorities tend to purchase social care services from other organisations, such as private and voluntary sector providers, whereas in England, they tend to purchase from their own statutory providers as well. In Northern Ireland there is GP funding, unlike in England where funding is mainly through NHS trusts.**

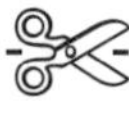

These questions guide you through the topic. If you need help to answer them, look at pages 28–31 of the Collins textbook.

7.5 short **questions** and **activities**

1 Why is the structure and organisation of care services in Northern Ireland harder to describe than those in other parts of the UK?

2 What is the full name of the DHSSPS in Northern Ireland? What are its three strategic aims?

3 Who is responsible for purchasing care services in Northern Ireland?

4 Explain what is meant by GP funding?

5 What is significant about the date 1999 in Scotland?

6 What is the responsibility of the regional health boards in Scotland?

7 In Scotland, which agencies, units or trusts are looked after by the health boards and by the local authorities?

summaryworksheet

NORTHERN IRELAND – NOW AND IN THE FUTURE

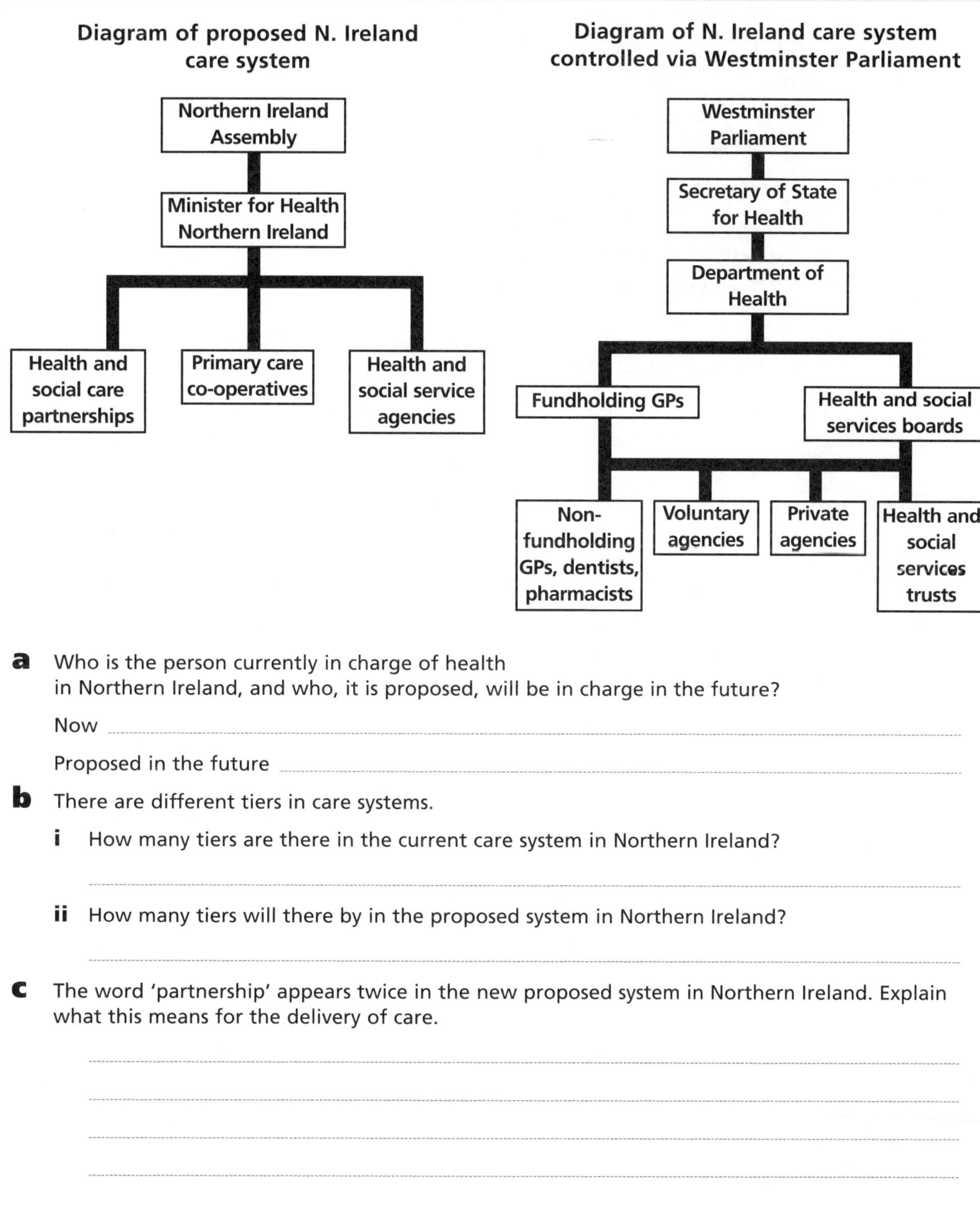

a Who is the person currently in charge of health in Northern Ireland, and who, it is proposed, will be in charge in the future?

Now ....

Proposed in the future ....

b There are different tiers in care systems.

i How many tiers are there in the current care system in Northern Ireland?

....

ii How many tiers will there by in the proposed system in Northern Ireland?

....

c The word 'partnership' appears twice in the new proposed system in Northern Ireland. Explain what this means for the delivery of care.

....

....

....

....

....

HOW WILL THINGS CHANGE?

a Here are some care workers in Northern Ireland:

- Patrick, a GP
- Marie, a private agency nurse
- Ross, a social worker

Outline the way each of them might work under the proposed new care system, compared to the present system controlled by the Westminster Parliament.

b Imagine that you have been elected Minister for Health, Northern Ireland. How would you ensure that the most vulnerable groups in Northern Ireland are catered for under the new proposals?

c Produce a booklet, suitable for a layperson, which illustrates the key changes that will take place under the proposed new care system under the Northen Ireland Assembly.

7.6 The private, voluntary and informal care sectors

It is important that students realise that care is provided in many different ways. This topic looks at the different sectors of independent and informal care provision. Students need to know that this type of care provision is non-statutory and in addition to the statutory care provision that they have met already. Some of the students may themselves be infomal carers or know someone who is an informal carer. Sensitivity should be exercised when discussing such topics.

The pictures in the *Getting you thinking* section show different aspects of care. The questions should stimulate discussion about the different sectors of care. This will be an opportunity to clear up any initial misconceptions about terms such as 'voluntary' and 'private'.

Answers to the *Check your understanding* questions on page 35 of the Collins textbook.

1 **Reasons for the increase in independent sector care provision over the last twenty years are: governments have encouraged that provision, the ageing population has demanded an increase in health and social care, there is a rise in the need for childcare with more women working, and there is a lack of public services in some areas.**

2 **The main characteristics of the private care sector are: it is provided on a commercial basis, with the practitioners working there operating to make a profit.**

3 **The main characteristics of the voluntary care sector are: their establishment (because a group of people decided to set it up – no law was required), they are usually registered charities and do not make a profit, and they are partly staffed and run by unpaid volunteers.**

4 **Informal carers are not professionally qualified, but look after relatives, friends or neighbours in their own homes. Many combine this with full-time paid employment. Informal carers provide the largest volume of care services in the UK, often filling 'gaps' in formal services. The formal care system would not be able to cope without them.**

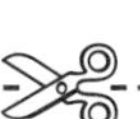

These questions guide you through the topic. If you need help to answer them, look at pages 32-35 of the Collins textbook.

7.6 short **questions** and **activities**

1. What does the independent sector comprise?
2. What type of health and care services are people now more willing to buy?
3. How many people in Britain are estimated to use private health of one kind or another? What are some of their reasons for doing this?
4. Give the three forms of private sector health and social care provision.
5. Explain what a 'philanthropic' person is. Give one example of such a person.
6. What is meant by the voluntary sector being a 'safety net'?
7. Make a list of the people who might be informal carers. For each person describe a range of care tasks they might carry out.

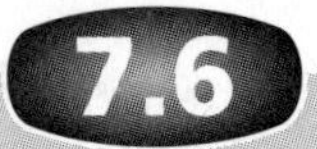

summary worksheet

THE DIFFERENT SECTORS OF CARE (INDEPENDENT AND INFORMAL)

Complete this summary table about the different sectors of care that are independent and informal.

	Private sector	*Voluntary sector*	*Informal sector*
Key characteristics			
Examples of who might work here			
Examples of who might receive care			
Examples of what services might be provided			
Advantages of this type of care			
Disadvantages of this type of care			

INFORMAL CARERS

The graph shows the percentage of informal carers, by age and sex, in England and Wales in 2001.

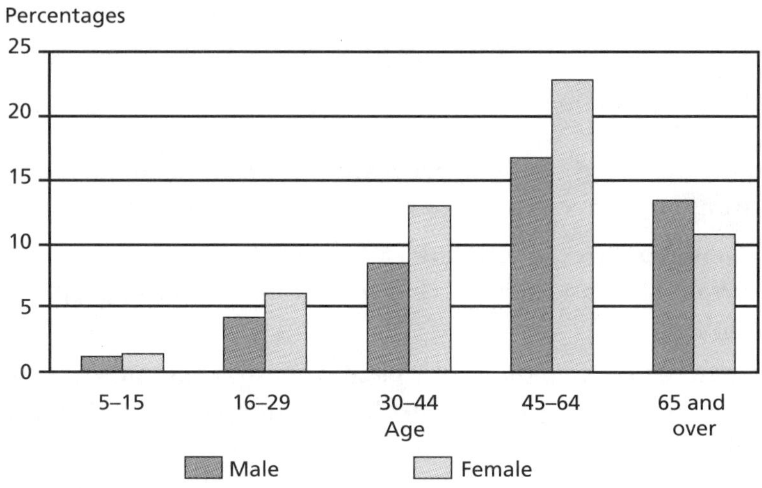

Carers: by age and sex, April 2001, England & Wales

a Write a short paragraph summarising the information shown in the graph.

b Suggest reasons for the profile of the informal carers.

c What other information would be needed to know the actual numbers of carers of each age group and sex?

7.7 Planning care for individual needs

Planning care for an individual's needs involves the use of a care plan cycle. Knowing the generic stages in the care plan cycle will enable students to think about care in a structured way. It will also enable them to answer examination questions more easily. It is important that the students realise that it is a cycle that can go round several times, depending on a client's changing needs. The importance of individualised care and involving clients is stressed.

There is a case study that runs through the topic. This illustrates well what happens in each of the stages. The *Getting you thinking* section introduces the students to the case study, and the questions should promote good discussion about what the students know and believe already, before studying the care plan cycle.

Answers to the *Check your understanding* questions on page 41 of the Collins textbook.

1 **The main stages of the care planning cycle are: assessing need, planning of care, implementation/intervention, monitoring and review/evaluation.**

2 **Care plans are evaluated to see whether care goals have been met and whether the current level and type of care provision remains appropriate for the individual.**

3 **Individualised care planning is thought to lead to better care practice than task-focused care delivery as it is more likely to address the specific needs of an individual.**

4 **Service users can be involved in the care planning cycle by asking them directly for their details at the assessment stage. They can be encouraged to take an active part in their own care provision and can provide valuable feedback when the plan is being monitored. They may also be involved at the review/evaluation stage, where they may be consulted about what they found helped and how their care needs may have changed.**

5 **Involving service users in their care planning increases the likelihood that the care plan will reflect their wishes and priorities. It also means that they are more likely to cooperate as the plans haven't been forced upon them.**

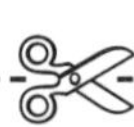

These questions guide you through the topic. If you need help to answer them, look at pages 36–41 of the Collins textbook.

7.7 short **questions** and **activities**

1. Why are members of a care team more likely to take a similar approach to their work than if they worked separately?
2. Describe briefly what is meant by 'task-focused' care. Give two disadvantages of this type of care.
3. List the four different sources of assessment information.
4. Describe in your own words the aims of a care plan.
5. Explain why someone might require a new assessment of needs.
6. List the different questions that should be asked when evaluating a care plan.
7. What is meant by the term 'empowerment'? How could empowerment of a service user be achieved?

summary worksheet

APPLICATION OF THE CARE PLAN CYCLE

You will need the case study about Tom Farmer (pages 38 and 39) for this worksheet.

Fill in the table to summarise what would happen in each part of the care plan cycle for Tom. You will need to go through the different parts of the case study and pick out some of the main points given.

Stage of the care plan cycle	*What happens in this part of the cycle for Tom*
Assessing need	
Care planning	
Implementation/ intervention	
Monitoring	
Review/ evaluation	

REVIEWING/EVALUATION CARE PLANS

Read the following case study and answer the questions that follow.

> Tyler is 19 years of age and was recently involved in a motorcycle accident. The left side of his body was damaged and he now has limited use of his left arm and leg. Tyler has had many operations and he has had to learn how to walk again. He had an assessment six months ago that recommended physiotherapy to help him improve the grip in his hand. He now finds that his grip is much improved. Tyler would like to move out of his parents' house and live by himself. Tyler has been invited to a review meeting with a social worker, occupational therapist and the phsyiotherapist.

a Why is it important that the physiotherapist is present at the review meeting?

b Describe how the change in Tyler's circumstances might affect the evaluation of Tyler's care plan and the current assessment of his needs.

c Why is it particularly important that Tyler is present at the review meeting?

d Write a short paragraph explaining what Tyler's care planning might involve now. Include the words 'normalisation', 'advocacy' and 'empowerment'.

7.8 Working in a care organisation

This topic looks at different types of care organisations from the point of view of their organisational structure and culture. The student is introduced to the advantages and disadvantages of each type, from the points of view of the person working there and the clients.

The data in the *Getting you thinking* section focuses the students on the NHS, and the questions allow them to consider the different types of people who work there. It would be interesting to ask the students if the information is consistent with what they knew or thought.

Answers to the *Check your understanding* questions on page 45 of the Collins textbook.

1 **The care sector that contains the largest number of carers in the UK is the statutory care sector, in particular the NHS.**

2 **A simple way of defining an organisation's culture is 'the way that the organisation does things'. This is reflected by the values and beliefs of the people who work there.**

3 **Two contrasting types of organisational culture are 'supporting and enabling' and 'formal, bureaucratic and rule-based'.**

4 **The type of culture may affect a care practitioner's decision-making process, management style, accountability, goals and objectives, and actions and behaviour. It is often the case that the culture of the organisation is so strong that the care practitioner's own decisions and actions may not be able to be expressed.**

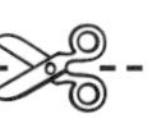

These questions guide you through the topic. If you need help to answer them, look at pages 42–45 of the Collins textbook.

7.8 short **questions** and **activities**

1. Summarise, in your own words, the ways in which an organisation expresses its culture.
2. What principle is Charles Handy's typology based on?
3. Explain what is meant by a democratic, participative and 'flat' structure in an organisation. What type of culture would this be most likely to be a feature of?
4. Name the four different organisational cultures identified in Charles Handy's typology.
5. Explain what is meant by a mission statement. Why is such a statement important?

summaryworksheet

DIFFERENT TYPES OF CULTURE

Charles Handy identified four different types of culture:

- The power culture
- The role culture
- The task culture
- The person culture.

a For each of the following descriptions, write down the culture it most applies to.

i The emphasis is on achieving definable results and getting things done.

....

ii A person's job title or position is central to their experience of the organisation.

....

iii If there is an organisational structure, it exists only to serve the individuals within it.

....

iv Influence spreads out from a central figure or group.

....

b Give one advantage and one disadvantage of a role culture.

Advantage ....

....

....

Disadvantage ....

....

....

c Give an example of where a task culture would work well.

....

....

WHICH KIND OF STRUCTURE AND CULTURE?

Read the following case study and answer the questions that follow.

> Mr Brown manages a small, private, residential care home for the elderly. There is no formal staffing structure and the ten care workers all have a similar status. Mr Brown arranges to meet with the care workers as often as he can. He encourages them to share information and concerns with him and with each other. Mr Brown says the motto of the care home is 'clients first'.

a Explain what type of organisation structure exists at the care home.

b Explain what type of culture exists at the care home. Discuss the advantages and disadvantages of this type of culture – for the people that work there and for the clients. What do you think might happen if Mr Brown left?

c Write a mission statement for the care home.

7.9 Quality assurance issues in care

It is very important the students understand that there are procedures for ensuring that the quality of care meets certain standards. The students are introduced to the idea of a national care policy and the key issues to focus on when trying to understand quality issues. The organisations and the people within organisations responsible for monitoring care are identified. The students should realise that care practitioners themselves play a large part in determining whether expected service standards are achieved.

The case study in the *Getting you thinking* section provides an opportunity for the students to realise that there is a need for quality assurance. The students will rightly be appalled that this could happen and the questions provide an opportunity for wider discussions about quality of care. It would be interesting to revisit questions 3 and 4 after the students have studied the topic to see if their answers are any different.

Answers to the *Check your understanding* questions on page 49 of the Collins textbook.

1 **Promoting or monitoring the quality of care services may be carried out through audits, assessing complaints, internal inspections or by using Total Quality Management.**

2 **The purpose of the National Service Frameworks is to set out principles and establish national standards of service provision for specific areas of practice.**

3 **In England the quality of public sector care services is monitored by the Healthcare Commission and the Commission for Social Care Inspection. In Northern Ireland the Health and Personal Social Services Regulation and Improvement Authority perform this role. In Scotland, the Scottish Commission for the Regulation of Care has this responsibility. In Wales, care standards and the quality of practice are inspected by the Care Standards Inspectorate for Wales.**

4 **Individual care practitioners are made accountable for the quality of their care practice through workplace supervision and monitoring of their practice, through the professional codes of practice and codes of conduct, and through the laws and legal duties they are subject to.**

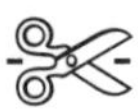

These questions guide you through the topic. If you need help to answer them, look at pages 46–49 of the Collins textbook.

7.9 short **questions** and **activities**

1 Outline the three key focuses that help the understanding of the quality assurance system.

2 Rewrite the definition of a quality service in your own words.

3 Briefly, what are the aims of (a) the Citizen's Charter and (b) the Patient's Charter?

4 List the key regulatory and standard-setting organisations in the UK.

5 What is meant by 'clinical governance'? Write one sentence outlining its importance.

6 Identify people who might monitor care standards.

7.9

summary worksheet

QUALITY ASSURANCE IN CARE

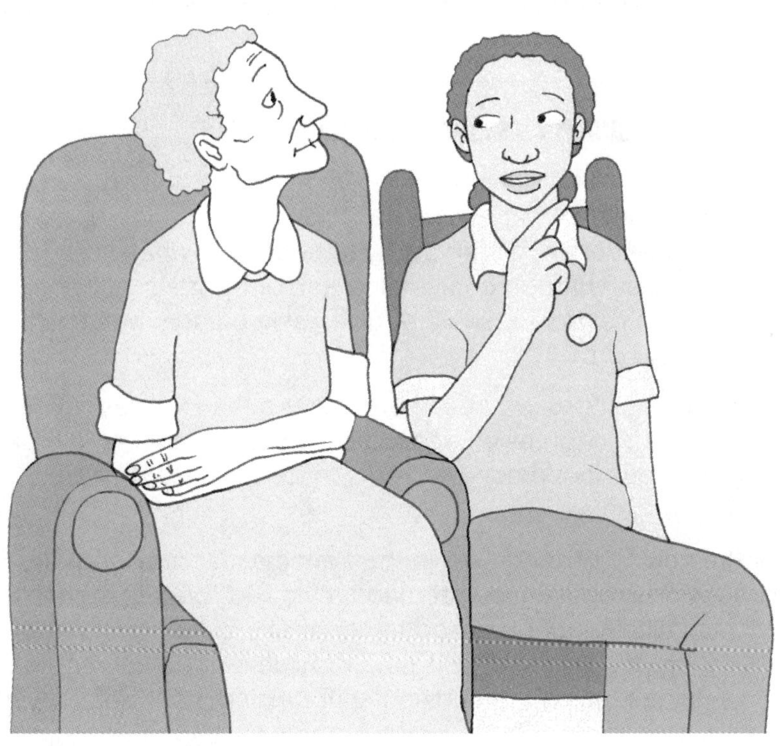

The patient shown in the picture lives in a residential care home.

a Explain how the information shown in the picture relates to the Patient's Charter.

b The care worker shown in the picture is accountable for the quality of her practice. Explain the ways in which this would happen.

c Explain why it is important that care services are inspected and regulated.

TRAINING CARE PRACTITIONERS

Read the following extract from a company that trains care practitioners, and answer the questions.

QUALITY ASSURANCE in care training

The principal aim of all our training is the increased well-being and improved quality of life for service users. This is achieved through improving staff confidence in their ability to cope with whatever situations might arise through challenging and/or aggressive behaviour, and through proactive techniques that give service users better control of their own behaviours.

Training staff in robust procedures to understand the people they work with and to deal with aggression and violence when it occurs is crucial to providing high-quality person-centred services for people with intellectual impairments.

It is also extremely important to have the systems that are used and all training procedures regularly audited and reviewed. We are developing training for staff who might be asked to undertake such a process by their organisation. We will be offering the providers of person-centred services this unique training in auditing staff training and related system procedures.

a In your own words, give the two ways in which the principal aim of the training is achieved.

b Explain what is meant by 'person-centred' services.

c Explain what is meant by 'auditing and reviewing' training procedures. Who might be involved in doing this?

d Discuss the statement, 'We don't need training procedures for our staff. We just ask them to be nice to the clients'.

Care professions in the NHS

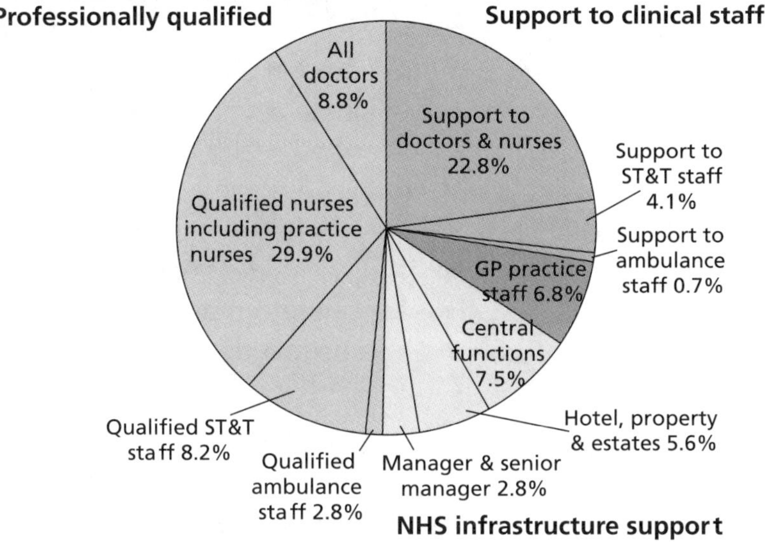

Number of staff in the NHS in 2004, DOH (2005)

Occupational group	Employed in NHS
Nursing, midwifery and health visiting	397,515
Doctors	117,036
Qualified scientific, therapeutic and technical (ST & T) staff	128,883
Qualified ambulance staff	17,272
NHS infrastructure support	211,489
GP Practice staff	90,110

The **Promoting Health and Well-being** unit is centred around a practical activity and will require the students to plan, implement and evaluate a small-scale health promotion. The topic can be drawn from any area relevant to health and social care but the target group should be from one of the following client groups – people who are ill, young children, older people or individuals with specific needs. Students will learn why health promotion campaigns are carried out and how topics and target groups are identified. They will study the different approaches to health education and how they are put into practice. Skills for delivering a health promotion activity will be developed through an understanding of the processes of planning, implementing and evaluating.

The health promotion activity should take approximately 15 hours to complete and may be carried out as part of a group. The unit will be assessed through an individual written report which will demonstrate the knowledge and understanding of the promotion of health and well-being and show evidence of the student's ability to conduct a small-scale health promotion. To achieve a good grade, students will need to demonstrate independent research skills, with information drawn from at least four sources of different types. They will also need to show an excellent ability to plan and implement their health promotion, an in-depth understanding of at least four health promotion models and approaches, and the use of a variety of media and materials. The report should indicate a good understanding of evaluation and give well-reasoned conclusions. Students should demonstrate a high level of independent thinking and initiative.

Promoting Health and Well-being

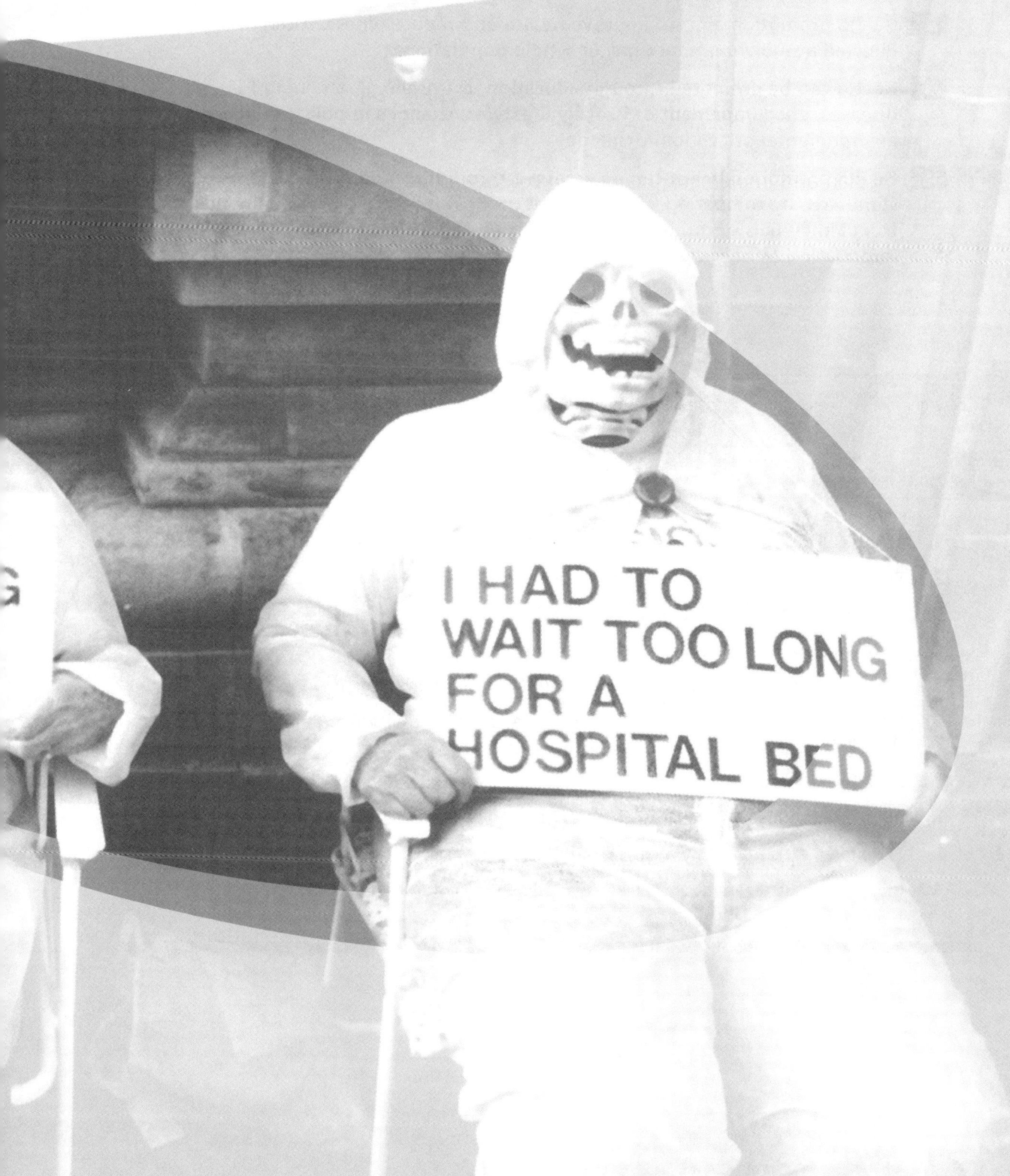

8.1 Why promote health and well-being?

Before considering how to promote health and well-being it is important to consider what is understood by 'health' and to explore the different aspects of health as applied to individuals and communities. Student should also examine the evidence that undertaking health promotion activities actually leads to an improvement in health. By looking at the familiar advice contained in the 'Ten tips for better health', links can be made to some well-advertised improvements in health that have occurred. The tension between the individual's responsibility for their own health and that of society can then be considered. Ideas such as understanding that knowledge of facts alone is not always sufficient to change health behaviour and that there are a number of different levels of health need are introduced.

Answers to the *Check your understanding* questions on page 55 of the Collins textbook.

1 **There are eight different aspects to an individual's health – physical, mental, emotional, spiritual, social, sexual, societal and environmental.**

2 **Health promotion aims to improve health and reduce illness. It can be directed at individuals, groups, or whole populations.**

3 **Health can be promoted through education, counselling, screening for diseases, encouragement of healthy lifestyles, changes in policy, or social, environmental or economic change.**

4 **Health promotion needs can be assessed through comparison with accepted standards, by comparing with different groups or responding to demands from individuals or groups. The starting point will always be to collect information to back-up any decision.**

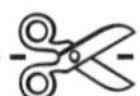

These questions guide you through the topic. If you need help to answer them, look at pages 52–55 of the Collins textbook.

8.1 short **questions** and **activities**

1. List the 'Ten tips for better health' from *Saving Lives – Our Healthier Nation*.
2. Explain what is meant by a 'holistic' view of health.
3. How did the WHO define health in 1946?
4. Write out your own definition of health promotion.
5. Explain the difference between 'primary,' 'secondary' and 'tertiary' health education.
6. Describe a health promotion that is aimed at an individual taking action to improve their own health.
7. Describe how environmental factors can affect an individual's health.
8. Identify two different health promotion campaigns aimed at the whole population.
9. Explain what is meant by a comparative need.
10. Identify the different sources of information that could be used to confirm the need for a health promotion.

summary worksheet

ASPECTS OF HEALTH

In the table below, the words and definitions of aspects of health are jumbled up. Match the correct definition to each word.

Aspect of health	*Definition*
Physical	An individual's beliefs and values; may include religious beliefs and practices; personal creeds; ways of peace of mind.
Mental	Ability to make and maintain relationships with other people.
Emotional	Functioning of the body.
Spiritual	Ability to think clearly and make judgements.
Social	Ability to recognise feelings, such as fear or anger, and express them appropriately. Ability to cope with stress and anxiety.
Sexual	The way individuals are treated within a society – through racism or other inequalities, for example.
Societal	Standard of physical environment in which individuals live, including housing, sanitation and pollution.
Environmental	Acceptance and expression of one's own sexuality.

What does being 'healthy' mean to you?

In column 1 identify what aspect or aspects of health are being described. In column 2 put into rank order the statements that are most important for you. Compare your answers with others.

Being healthy means	1 Aspect of health	2 Rank of importance to me
1 Being physically fit		
2 Being a non-smoker		
3 Feeling happy most of the time		
4 Getting on well with my friends		
5 Not getting stressed		
6 Taking exercise regularly		
7 Feeling comfortable with myself		
8 Not taking regular medication		
9 Being able to adapt easily to different situations		
10 Living in a 'good' neighbourhood		
11 Having personal beliefs and values		
12 Living a long life		
13 Having a 'good' diet		
14 Being able to relax		

extension**activity**sheet

SAVING LIVES – OUR HEALTHIER NATION

Saving Lives – Our Healthier Nation was published in1999. You will find a copy in the library or on the internet at http://www.official-documents.co.uk

a Complete the following statement which is in Chapter 1:

Saving Lives – Our Healthier Nation is an action plan for ....

and .... in England, especially

....

b For one of the four priority areas of cancer, coronary heart disease and strokes, accidents, and mental health, use the document to investigate in detail the following:

i How well the UK death rates compare with other countries in Western Europe

ii The main causes of death and disease in the category

iii The main actions that are planned by the health services

iv The main actions that individuals should take

v The partnerships that are suggested in order to improve health.

Identifying health and well-being issues

The previous topic introduced the concept that a health promotion is usually developed in response to an identified need or priority. An example is given of the need to protect children from the sun. Here, the factual basis for these priorities is explored by examining a number of ways in which health needs are reported. Epidemiological data is illustrated, including the sources, analysis, formats and application of research findings. Additional research and discussion of appropriate health-related findings would give further opportunities to apply this aspect of the unit. Targets for health and well-being are discussed with reference to both national and international targets. There is an opportunity to make comparisons between the UK and countries from the developing world. Other strategies, guidelines or reasons for health promotion are introduced, demonstrating the breadth of influences on any target-setting and suggesting that there are many more areas for further research.

Answers to the *Check your understanding* questions on page 61 of the Collins textbook.

1 **Epidemiology studies the patterns of disease and illness. Findings from epidemiological studies will therefore provide information on the health of a population, and the causes and risk factors linked with ill-health, and indicate where there are possibilities for making improvements through health promotion.**

2 **The national targets in Saving Lives – Our Healthier Nation are, by 2010:**
- **To reduce the death rate from cancer in people under 75 by at least a fifth.**
- **To reduce the death rate from coronary heart disease and stroke and related diseases in people under 75 by at least two fifths.**
- **To reduce the death rate from accidents by at least a fifth and reduce the rate of serious injury from accidents by at least a tenth.**
- **To reduce the death rate from suicide and undetermined injury by at least a fifth.**

Health promotion can play a vital part in meeting these targets as it can influence individuals and communities to adopt healthier lifestyles. Many of the causes of these aspects of ill-health are to do with lifestyle choices such as smoking, alcohol, drugs, diet and exercise. Other risk factors can be mitigated through greater public awareness of preventative measures such as screening programmes and health and safety measures.

3 **In 2000 the UN published its Millennium Development Goals, most of which are health-related. Poverty, hunger and diseases such as HIV/AIDS and malaria are all linked to health, as are the goals to reduce child mortality and improve maternal health. The target of universal primary education allows individuals to learn about health and how they can care for themselves, their families and communities, while the goal to promote gender equality and empower women would lead to women having better life experiences and greater influence over their own health and the health of their children. The broader aspect of environmental sustainability and global partnership tackles the wider concept of more equal distribution of wealth and protection of the environment.**
Students may also find targets that have been set by other international bodies such as the World Health Organization in eradicating smallpox and eliminating polio in the Global Polio Eradication Initiative. There are also targets for health set by the EU.

4 **Other reasons may include an outbreak of an infectious disease such as meningitis; an area of public concern; new scientific discoveries; or media interest.**

These questions guide you through the topic. If you need help to answer them, look at pages 56-61 of the Collins textbook.

8.2 short**questions**and**activities**

1. Identify four sources of statistical data which provide information on the health of the population.
2. Identify two advantages of using health status data when planning a health promotion.
3. Identify two areas of health in the UK that are not included in the national targets but have separate strategies. What are the main aims of the strategies?
4. Explain the term' National Service Framework'.
5. Why may individuals in the UK need to know about health in other parts of the world?
6. Identify two infectious diseases that are common in the UK for which there are health promotion programmes.
7. Describe a new scientific discovery that has influenced health promotion.

8.2

summaryworksheet

1 UNDERSTANDING DATA

Look at four examples of health status data that are available online (see suggested sources below). For each example, explain which groups (male/female, age, ethnic group, geographical area) are most at risk and how health promotion activities could be targeted to address the problems.

Suggested sources

- In Saving Lives (http://www.official-documents.co.uk) there are charts showing:

1 UK having the highest rate of live births to teenage girls in Europe and a map of which local authorities have the highest rates (Figs 9.1 and 9.2).

2 Accident rates increase as children grow up (Fig 7.4).

3 Survival rate for cancer better in affluent areas than in deprived areas (Fig 5.6).

4 Women in some ethnic groups have low uptake of potentially life-saving cervical cancer smears (Fig 9.8).

- Dr Foster (www.drfoster.co.uk) has data showing inequalities in health experience.

2 CURRENT CONCERNS

Review health-related stories in the media during the last week. This could be in newspapers, magazines or the storyline in a 'soap' on television or radio. What health concerns are currently being discussed and why?

Choose two issues and analyse the implications for health promotion for each:

a Is it already part of a health promotion or a new issue?

b Is the coverage positive or negative?

c How has the media interest supported the promotion of health?

d How could the promotion of the specific health issue be further developed through the media?

COMPARING COUNTRIES

Choose either Kenya or India and compare with the UK.

1 Find out some basic facts about your chosen country and the UK such as:

- The size of the population
- The life expectancy
- The number of doctors per head of population
- The average income.

2 Find out the major causes of death and disease in each country:

3 Now consider how the diseases that you have identified are caused and how they are treated. What measures might be available in each country to help control disease?

4 Find out the figures of child mortality – why do you think they are different?

5 The UK has a clean water supply and effective sanitation – what difference does that make to the health of the population?

6 What would you do? Suggest which health needs would be prioritised in each country.

8.3 Health promotion agencies

The ranges of people and organisations that may influence health are explored, including the possibility of both formal and informal settings. The idea that cooperation between agencies and groups may be required in order to achieve a successful outcome is discussed. Within the major groupings of different agencies that have a link with health, examples are given and their role explored – but many other suggestions could be offered in the light of personal or local experiences. The influence of the mass media is highlighted and the opportunity for wide-ranging topical debate about their role could be developed.

Answers to the *Check your understanding* questions on page 65 of the Collins textbook.

1 **Health promotion is rarely the responsibility of one agency working on its own. Because so many different factors can influence an individual's health, there may need to be several different solutions. For example, an individual trying to give up smoking may have the help of a health professional but will find it easier if his workplace is non-smoking and the cost of cigarettes is increased.**

2 **The NHS is a major agency for promoting health. It tackles disease and illness but also seeks to prevent ill-health through early intervention such as through regular screening programmes. Health professionals give advice about healthy living in a variety of settings including primary care, the community and hospitals.**

3 **Choice of three from the following:**
International organisations National governmental organisations
Local government Voluntary organisations and pressure groups
Commercial organisations Work-related Mass media.

4 **The mass media can convey health promotion messages through articles, features, advertisements, press releases or storylines in programmes. These are very powerful ways of raising awareness about health but they may have positive or negative effects, depending on the way in which the issue is reported.**

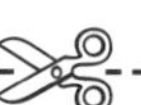

These questions guide you through the topic. If you need help to answer them, look at pages 62–65 of the Collins textbook.

8.3 short**questions**and**activities**

1. Explain how health can be promoted informally.
2. What is meant by a 'healthy alliance'? Suggest what sort of organisations might take part.
3. List the health professionals that are members of the Primary Health Care Team and explain how they can promote health.
4. How are local authorities involved in promoting health?
5. Identify a voluntary organisation that may promote the health of older people.
6. What is a pressure group? Identify one that is linked to health.
7. Describe how commercial organisations may become involved in promoting health.
8. How are employers responsible for promoting the health of their employees?
9. Describe one message about health that has been promoted through the mass media.

summaryworksheet

ORGANISATIONS PROMOTING HEALTH

Review the statements below from three agencies and identify how and why each of these organisations can be seen as promoting health. Which aspects of health might they specifically promote? Do they work towards any national targets?

Royal Society for the Prevention of Accidents

RoSPA's mission is to enhance the quality of life by exercising a powerful influence for accident prevention. It is a registered charity which aims to campaign for change, influence opinion, contribute to debate, educate and inform – for the good of all. By providing information, advice, resources and training, RoSPA is actively involved in the safety and prevention of accidents in all areas of life – at work, in the home, on the roads, in schools, at leisure, and on (or near) water.

Samaritans

Samaritans is available 24 hours a day to provide confidential emotional support for people who are experiencing feelings of distress or despair, including those which may lead to suicide.

Samaritans' vision is for a society in which fewer people die by suicide, people are able to explore their feelings, and people are able to acknowledge and respect the feelings of others.

NSPCC

The NSPCC's mission is to end cruelty to children. Our vision is a society in which all children are loved, valued and able to fulfil their potential. In other words, a society that will not tolerate child abuse – whether sexual, physical, emotional or neglect.

extension**activity**sheet

RESEARCHNG ONE ORGANISATION

Find the mission statement and values of one organisation and identify how and why it promotes health.

The organisation

Type of agency: ....

Mission statement, including target group: ....

....

Values: ....

....

How the organisation promotes health

An example of one health promotion activity that the organisation has undertaken:

....

The specific aim of the activity: ....

....

How successful do you think the promotion proved to be, and why?

....

....

8.4 Approaches to health promotion

Although there may be agreement about the need for health promotion, different individuals and organisations may take very different attitudes and approaches to the solution. The choice of approach will depend on a number of factors including the priority put on different aspects of health. The example gives an opportunity to explore the possible different approaches by a number of individuals or groups. This gives an insight into the five major approaches which provide the basis for most health promotion activity. Other reasons for the choice of approach, such as the availability of resources, are also introduced, and will be further developed when considering the practical application to the health promotion activity which is part of this unit.

Answers to the *Check your understanding* questions on page 71 of the Collins textbook.

1

Model	Aim	Activity
Medical	Reduce medically defined disease and disability	Medical intervention to high-risk groups or populations
Behaviour change	Individuals to adopt a healthy lifestyle	Activities aimed at changing attitudes and behaviours
Educational	Individuals to acquire knowledge, understanding and skills to make and act upon informed decisions	Giving of information. Exploration of attitudes to health. Development of skills such as decision-making
Client-centred empowerment	Clients to identify own health needs	Facilitate the identification of needs and work with clients to develop their knowledge and skills
Societal change	Change physical and socio-economic environment to support health lifestyles	Political and social action, including legislation to improve environment for healthy living

2 **Smoking would be discouraged using an educational approach when the health promoter gave the smoker information about the dangers of smoking, for example the risks of heart and respiratory disease. Attitudes to smoking would be explored by discussing whether the smoker's friends or family smoked and their attitude to the situation. Skills needed to resist pressure to smoke or to stop smoking would be developed. The decision not to smoke would be left to the client, once they had received all the information.**

3 **Participation in exercise could be increased through societal change by making participation in exercise easier. This could be by an increase in sports facilities, an increase in sports in schools, and subsidised rates for exercise classes.**

4 **The health of children is promoted throughout their life from the health services, schools, youth clubs and societies as well as by commercial companies. Examples from each category of approach can be illustrated : medical – through regular screening throughout pregnancy, early childhood including immunisation programme; behaviour change – children are influenced to change certain unhealthy behaviours, such as poor hygiene practices or unhealthy eating; educational – children are educated about health throughout their schooldays, including about drugs, smoking, etc.; client-centred – as children get older they may themselves identify areas of health that are important to them, and make their own decisions; societal change – children will frequently be affected by changes in the physical or socio-economic environment – for example, the retaining of school playing fields, expanding sports facilities, the introduction of healthy school meals, the removal of 'unhealthy drinks' machines.**

These questions guide you through the topic. If you need help to answer them, look at pages 66–71 of the Collins textbook.

8.4 short **questions** and **activities**

1. What factors need to be considered when deciding which would be the most appropriate approach for a health promotion?
2. Describe what is meant by a medical model of health promotion and give two examples of the model in practice.
3. Identify two weaknesses of the behaviour change model.
4. How are the aims of the educational model put into practice?
5. Explain why the values of the client-centred model differ from the other approaches to health promotion.
6. Identify two advantages of the societal change model.
7. Why is it important to know what skills are required for a specific promotion?
8. How would the choice of target group affect the choice of health promotion approach?
9. Why might the medical model need more resources than other approaches?

8.4

summary worksheet

1 APPROACHES TO HEALTH PROMOTION

Complete this table

	Aim	Activity	Values	Strengths	Weaknesses
Medical	Reduce medically defined disease and disability		Patients' compliance with the experts		• Authoritarian • Relies on infrastructure to support programme, e.g. screening • People need to be persuaded to use facilities
Behaviour change	Individuals to adopt a healthy lifestyle			• Encourages personal change • Not imposed by others • Appeals to the 'adult' in a person	• Behaviour not easy to change • Client susceptible to other influences • Intentions not always followed through
Educational	Individuals to acquire knowledge, understanding and skills to make and act upon informed decisions	Giving of information. Exploration of attitudes to health. Development of skills such as decision-making	The rights of informed individuals to choose is respected		
Client-centred empowerment	Clients to identify own health needs		Clients as equals. Clients are self-empowered to challenge and change	• Greater engagement of clients with own choice of topic. • Better outcomes through self-empowerment	
Societal change		Political and social action, including legislation to improve environment for healthy living		• Healthy behaviour becomes more acceptable • Reaches a wide group of people • Some healthy behaviours become law	• Social rebels may oppose change • A range of approaches needed to effect social change • Needs a large-scale approach

2 AIMS AND ACTIVITIES

Taking smoking as an example, identify the aims and activities that would take place under each approach:

	Aim	Activity
Medical	Freedom from lung disease, heart disease and other smoking-related diseases	
Behaviour change		Persuasive education to prevent non-smokers from starting and to persuade smokers to give up
Educational		
Client-centred empowerment		
Societal change		

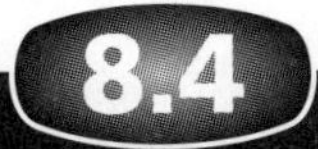

extension**activity**sheet

ANALYSING TWO HEALTH PROMOTIONS

Fill in the following, once you have chosen two health promotions to analyse.

First health promotion activity

Name of the health promotion ....

Which model/approach was used? ....

Why was this model/approach used? ....

....

Was this an appropriate model/approach to use? Why/why not? ....

....

....

Which professionals were involved? ....

....

What resources were used? ....

....

....

What were the results of the health promotion? ....

....

....

Second health promotion activity

Name of the health promotion ....

Which model/approach was used? ....

Why was this model/approach used? ....

....

Was this an appropriate model/approach to use? Why/why not? ....

....

....

Which professionals were involved? ....

....

What resources were used? ....

....

....

What were the results of the health promotion? ....

....

....

8.5 Health promotion methods and media

The choice of which form of media and which method to use for a health promotion is very important. The factors that influence that choice are explored, together with the principles on which the choice should be made. The appropriateness to the target group is discussed. An analysis of different examples of health promotion campaigns will demonstrate the wide variety of methods and their application. Choice of tone and style is seen as just as important as the method, such as whether to use leaflets or a TV advert. The advantages and disadvantages of using the mass media are identified. The application of knowledge gained from this topic will also support the development of the required health promotion activity.

Answers to the *Check your understanding* questions on page 77 of the Collins textbook.

1 **The factors are: the appropriateness of the resource for use with the target group; the characteristics of the group and what would be most suitable; whether issues of equality and diversity are considered; the accuracy of any information; the clarity of the information; the style and format; and the link with the aim of the promotion.**

2 **Health promotion should be seen to apply principles of equality and non-discrimination, despite the fact that studies show that certain groups are more vulnerable to certain diseases than others. Stereotyping should be avoided, and diversity should be celebrated through positive images of different physical cultural and social differences.**

3 **Leaflets/handouts can be used to give information and to support a presentation. The information can be taken away for future referral, shared with others and give greater detail, e.g. statistics. Handouts are easily produced. Posters can be used to raise awareness, can convey information, have high impact through challenging images and can be made cheaply. Presentations can be used to convey information to an audience, can be tailored to a specific group, go at the pace of the group, and use a range of methods to keep the audience attentive.**

4 **Advantages of using mass media: raises awareness about health issues; puts health on the public agenda effecting societal change; increases knowledge; influences attitude and behaviour change; has immediate emotional effect. Disadvantages of using mass media: responses may be short term; cannot convey complex information; cannot teach skills; may only change attitudes or behaviours if in combination with other enabling factors; some mass media stories may convey negative messages about health promotion.**

8.5 short **questions** and **activities**

1. What is meant by the characteristics of a group?
2. Give an example of a health promotion message that is only targeted at men, and one that is only targeted at women. Explain why these promotions are only targeted at one sex.
3. What is meant by using 'fear' tactics? When have they been used? Explain one advantage and one disadvantage of this approach.
4. Describe how the mass media is used by health promotion campaigns to raise awareness.
5. What part does the mass media play in informing the public about health behaviours of individuals? Identify a current story featuring an individual and their health behaviour.
6. How and when does the mass media promote unhealthy products and habits?
7. Describe sponsorship and its relationship to health.
8. When might a presentation be the most appropriate way of giving information that will promote health?
9. What are the disadvantages of using posters to convey health promotion messages?

summaryworksheet

GETTING THE LANGUAGE RIGHT

The extract below is a quote from 1603 by James I, King of England. Identify what habit he was describing, and put his message into language that would be suitable today.

> **'A custom, loathsome to the eye, hateful to the Nose, harmful to the Braine, dangerous to the Lungs, and in the black stinking fume thereof, nearest resembling the horrible Stygian smoke of the pit that is bottomless. By immoderate taking, the wealth of a great number of people is impaired, and their bodies unfit for labour.'**

GETTING THE IMAGE RIGHT

In 1986 and 1987 a major campaign was launched by the government in response to the rise in AIDS cases. It included a leaflet that was delivered to all households depicting an iceberg. The slogan was 'Don't die of ignorance' What interpretations could there have been of this slogan? What was it trying to convey?

DEFINITIONS

The following are medical terms that are in common usage. Find out what they mean and write down their definitions: AIDS; Cirrhosis; Dyspepsia; Mammogram; MMR; Osteoporosis; Podiatry; Prophylactic; Quarantine; Rhinitis; Sinusitis; Syndrome.

MEDIA COVERAGE

Choose a health-related topic (for example, alcohol, exercise, diet) and complete the table below about how it is currently portrayed in the media. Identify whether the coverage has a broadly positive or negative effect on health.

Type of mass media	*Description*
National or regional health promotion campaign using the mass media, e.g. advertisements	
Promotion of products by commercial organisations using health link	
Discussions or reports on the chosen topic	
Indirectly addressed in programmes, e.g. in storylines	
Behaviour related to topic by personalities	
Advertising of 'unhealthy' product	
Sponsorship	

extension**activity**sheet

TWO HEALTH PROMOTION CAMPAIGNS

Choose any two promotion campaigns, one of which has used the mass media. Analyse each one for its content, style, target group and likely impact, and fill in the following table.

HEALTH PROMOTION CAMPAIGN, USING THE MASS MEDIA	HEALTH PROMOTION CAMPAIGN, NOT USING THE MASS MEDIA
Description of content	**Description of content**
Style or format of promotion	**Style or format of promotion**
Target group	**Target group**
Expected impact	**Expected impact**
Success of the methods used	**Success of the methods used**

8.6 Ethical issues in health promotion

Building on the previous topics, it is obvious that different individuals will take differing views about promoting health. The ethical issues that surround health promotion do not necessarily have an obvious answer but provide a rich opportunity for discussion. Debates about such topics as individual choice, community good, informed choice, cost effectiveness, political control or sponsorship are linked with an understanding of the inequalities that exist in health. Examples of ethical dilemmas can be taken from case studies or from past or current health promotions. [There are a number of good illustrations of inequalities by social class, gender and international comparison in *Saving Lives – Our Healthier Nation*.]

Answers to the *Check your understanding* questions on page 81 of the Collins textbook.

1 **Informed choice ensures that an individual knows all the facts about the situation and is confident to express their own mind before being asked to make a choice. In health promotion, an individual's personal choice may not always meet the aims of the health promoter.**

2 **Victim blaming is when an individual is blamed for their own ill-health. In health promotion, the fact that some people do not wish to follow health advice may lead to a worsening of their health status.**

3 **Sponsorship of health promotion activities can bring in much-needed financial and other resources. The disadvantages are that the health promoter may be seen as endorsing a particular product and the independent credibility may be lost.**

4 **Inequalities in society have major effects on health. Income, education, housing and social exclusion all exercise profound influences on individuals and have been shown to cause physical, mental and social health problems.**

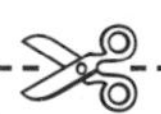

These questions guide you through the topic. If you need help to answer them, look at pages 78–81 of the Collins textbook.

8.6 short **questions** and **activities**

1. Why might a health promoter want the clients to 'comply' with advice rather than exercise 'informed choice'?
2. Give an example of a situation when a patient might be 'blamed' for their condition.
3. How might the cost-effectiveness of a screening programme be assessed?
4. Give an example of a change in advice about how to remain healthy or safe.
5. Why may national governments have an interest in health promotion?
6. What is a 'vested interest' and how might it affect health?
7. Why are health professionals expected to live a healthy lifestyle?
8. Explain how one of the major inequalities in society can affect an individual's health.
9. List the ethical principles that must be adhered to when undertaking research.

ETHICAL DILEMMAS

Look at the following situations. Identify what ethical dilemmas they pose for health promoters, and discuss your findings in your class.

1 Parents, pupils or staff at a school may wish to know of the presence of any HIV-positive child or member of staff. They may argue that it could be a possible health risk or that they could provide better care and support for the individual. Should they be told?

2 Immunisation is only effective if a high level of immunity is achieved in the population. Is it ethical for individuals to be persuaded to take up the vaccine against their wishes?

3 In 2005 George Best died at the age of 59. He had been an outstanding footballer and was admired by many young people. He was an alcoholic, and was diagnosed with cirrhosis of the liver, for which he had a transplant in 2002. He continued to drink until his death. What ethical dilemmas for health professionals does his story illustrate?

SCREENING

The following are facts about the screening process:

- Screening is never wholly routine and inclusive. It is targeted at risk groups and is usually age-related.
- Screening is spaced because of economic reasons and therefore individuals may develop the disease in the gaps between screening.
- The process may cause anxiety.
- The process may be uncomfortable, painful or risky.
- There may be false results.

Is screening always of benefit to everybody?

INEQUALITIES IN HEALTH

The chart shows evidence of inequalities in health.

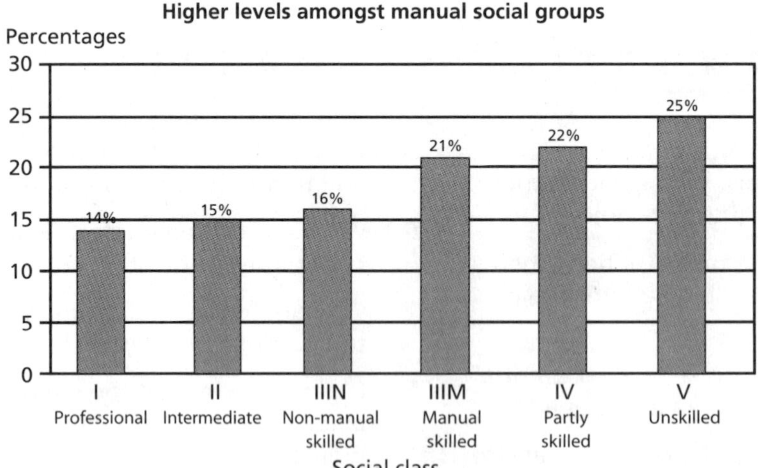

Obesa (Body Mass Index over 30). England 1996, woman aged 16 and over

Saving Lives – Our Healthier Nation

Social and Community Planning Research, Dept of Epidemiology and Public Health, Prescott-Clarke, P., Primatesta P eds

Health Survey for England, 1996, London: The Stationery Office 1998.

What health problems can obesity cause? Why might those in classes IV and V have such a significant difference in their levels of obesity? How might health promotion address inequalities in health?

HEALTH PROMOTION AND SPONSORSHIP

Choose two health promotion campaigns that have sponsorship – you could look for leaflets in your supermarket or the doctor's surgery, or you may see companies endorsing campaigns such as breast-awareness. Describe the health promotion and then answer the following questions:

1 Who is the sponsor? What are they best known for?

2 What link has the sponsor got with the promotion that they are sponsoring?

3 Does the fact that the sponsor is linked with health help their image in the eyes of the public?

4 For this health promotion, what are the specific advantages and disadvantages of being sponsored?

5 What are your own views about the campaign and its sponsorship?

PRESS STORIES ABOUT HEALTH

Review two recent press stories about health, and answer the following questions for each:

1 Summarise the story and identify its source.

2 Is the story covered in more than one part of the press? Is there any difference in the coverage? If so, what difference?

3 Are there any ethical issues arising from the topic of the story? Describe the issues, or explain why there are no issues.

4 Are there any ethical issues in the way in which the topic is reported? Explain the way in which it is reported.

Planning and preparing for a health promotion activity

The main emphasis is on the principles of planning and preparing for a health promotion activity. The application to planning for the assessed health promotion activity should be kept in mind throughout the study of the topic. The opening exercise is an opportunity to reflect on the difficulties of not planning ahead and getting caught up in a reactive process over which one has no control. The stages of the flowchart for planning and evaluation provide a summary of the main steps required while preparing a health promotion. Each stage is then explored in greater depth.

Answers to the *Check your understanding* questions on page 85 of the Collins textbook.

1
- **Identify consumers/clients/patients and their characteristics**
- **Identify consumer needs**
- **Decide on goals for health education**
- **Formulate specific objectives**
- **Identify resources**
- **Plan content and method in detail**
- **Plan evaluation methods**
- **Implement your plan**
- **Evaluate.**

2 **Smart objectives have the following characteristics**
Specific – clearly defined
Measurable – able to be quantified
Achievable – able to be completed
Realistic – appropriate to the circumstances
Timescale – able to set timings for completion.

3

Aim	Appropriate methods
Raising awareness of health issues	• Talks • Group work • Mass media • Displays • Campaigns
Providing information and improving knowledge	• One-to-one teaching • Group teaching • Written material • Displays • Mass media • Campaigns
Empowering: improving self-awareness, self-esteem, decision making	• Group work • Social skills training • Role play • Assertiveness training • Counselling
Changing attitudes, behaviour and lifestyles of individuals	• Group work • Skills training • Self-help groups • Advice • Group or individual work
Societal change: changing the physical or social environment	• Pressure groups • Lobbying • Community development • Planning and policy making • Legislation

Adapted from Ewles and Simnet, *Promoting Health: A Practical Guide*, Scutari Press, 1992.

4 **Methods of evaluation include the following:**
• 'Before and after' questioning, using questionnaires, interviews, discussions, written tests
• Observation of changes in attitudes and behaviours
• Changes in demand for health information
• Records of changes in health status, e.g. weight, blood pressure
• Analysis of interest in media coverage
• Measuring changes in environment
• Noting policy changes promoting 'healthy living', e.g. restriction on smoking, increased leisure facilities.

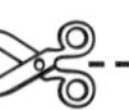

These questions guide you through the topic. If you need help to answer them, look at pages 82–85 of the Collins textbook.

8.7 short **questions** and **activities**

1. Explain why it is important to plan prior to commencing a health promotion.
2. What factors need to be taken into account when planning a health promotion?
3. Explain the difference between an aim and an objective.
4. Describe the range of resources that may be needed in order to carry out a health promotion.
5. Identify which methods would be most appropriate when aiming to change attitudes and behaviours.
6. Explain what 'empowering' individuals means and how it may be undertaken.
7. When might pressure groups be used, and how?
8. Give two reasons for undertaking an evaluation after the event.
9. Describe two types of evaluation, including one that is most appropriate for assessing small-scale promotions.

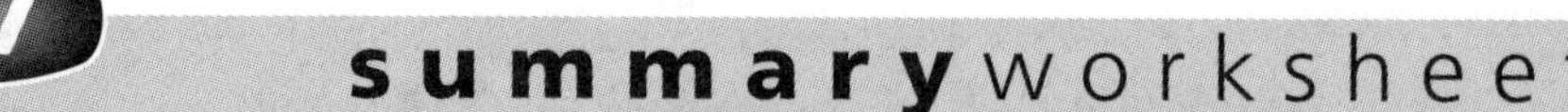

8.7 summary worksheet

FILL IN THE GAPS: AIMS AND METHODS IN HEALTH PROMOTION

Aim	Appropriate methods
.... of health issues	• Talks • Group work • Mass media • Displays • Campaigns
Providing information and improving knowledge	• One-to-one teaching • .... • Written material • .... • Mass media • Campaigns
.... : improving self-awareness, self-esteem, decision making	• Group work • Social skills training • Role play • .... • Counselling
Changing attitudes, behaviour and	• Group work • Skills training • .... • Advice • Group or individual work
Societal change: changing the physical or social environment	• Pressure groups • .... • Community development • Planning and policy making • ....

Adapted from Ewles and Simnet, *Promoting Health: A Practical Guide*, Scutari Press, 1992.

RESOURCES

Using a 'mind map', identify all the resources that are available to you, that you will need to undertake a health promotion.

PLANNING NATIONAL NO-SMOKING DAY

Using this table, plan a health promotion for the National No-Smoking Day in your local area – imagining that you are in charge!

The target group and their characteristics	*e.g. Smokers in the local further education college*
Needs of target group regarding smoking	
Goals of health promotion	
Specific objectives for activity	
The resources that will be needed	
Content, method of activity	
How it will be evaluated	

8.8 Carrying out a health promotion activity

This topic is about health promotion in action. As has already been considered, there will be many different forms of action – some of which will be appropriate, while others will not be so successful. Opportunities for discussion about the relevance and influence of specific types of action can be developed from examples – and then used to apply to proposals for the planned health promotion. The detailed considerations of team working, time management, resource allocation and planning around the physical factors can then be developed. Discussions about communication also link to principles covered in Unit 2, such as barriers to communication.

Answers to the *Check your understanding* questions on page 91 of the Collins textbook.

1 **An action plan should identify who will do what by when, and with what resources.**

2 **A decision needs to be made at the beginning as to whether it is to be an individual or group project. If it is to be a group activity then the roles of the different members should be clear.**

3 **Time is a resource that should be used efficiently and cost-effectively.**

4 **As well as the content of the health promotion, communication methods and physical factors – such as the room or other venue – need to be considered.**

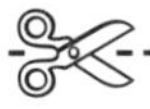

These questions guide you through the topic. If you need help to answer them, look at pages 86–91 of the Collins textbook.

8.8 short **questions** and **activities**

1 Describe the advantages and disadvantages of working as an individual.

2 List the characteristics of a successful team.

3 What preliminary stages may need to be undertaken before starting the planning to ensure that the activity can take place?

4 What are the two aspects of time management?

5 Give two tips for improving time management.

6 Describe two barriers to good communication that might exist.

7 What physical factors need to be taken into consideration before commencing the health promotion?

8 Describe the benefits of having a lesson plan for a presentation.

8.8 **summary**worksheet

FILL IN THE GAPS

An action plan is ....

Time management means ....

Communication is .... but there may be .... factors that restrict or .... the effectiveness. These are known as .... to communication. Examples are ....

....

One of the skills in good communication is active listening which is the process ....

....

....

My own plans for improving my time management are ....

....

....

....

MY ACTION PLAN

Break down the project into milestones or key events, indicating when certain things should happen and who is responsible for the action.

What needs to be done	By whom	By when	With what resource

extension**activity**sheet

PRIORITIES AND TIME ALLOCATION

a List the three goals/objectives – the tasks that you hope to complete – that are most important. They may be college-based or home-based.

Goal/Objective	*To be completed by*	*Time you have set aside*
1		
2		
3		

b Does your time allocation reflect the time needed to meet your goals?

Goal 1
Goal 2
Goal 3

c What other commitments need to be fitted in to your schedule?

My commitments	Time needed

d Now review your typical day

Activities	*Hours*
Sleeping	
Dressing	
Meals, including preparation and clearing up	
Family commitments	
Socialising	
Relaxing, TV/videos, etc.	
Exercise/Sport	
Travel	
Lessons	
Studying	
Work	
Other	
Other	
Total	*24*

e How much spare time have you got? Now put this into a weekly chart to show how you managed each day, highlighting when you were working towards the goals you have identified.

f Review how you worked towards your goals. Did you complete them in good time or were they rushed at the last moment? Rewrite your weekly schedule to ensure that your goals are completed.

8.9 Analysing and evaluating a health promotion activity

Evaluation is an integral part of any health promotion but the methods for gaining meaningful results need careful consideration. A vague and unfocused evaluation will lack clarity. Involving the individual who was responsible for undertaking the health promotion has advantages and disadvantages – they will have greater knowledge of the participants/circumstances etc., but they may not be so objective in their evaluation. The principles of successful evaluation are explored, and emphasis is given to the development of questionnaires which are the most common form of evaluation used in small-scale activities. Finally, guidance on writing of the report is given.

Answers to the *Check your understanding* questions on page 97 of the Collins textbook.

1 **Process evaluation** notes reactions to the activity, and identifies other factors affecting the activity, using interviews, diaries and observation. It involves participants and reviews responses from the particular target group. **Impact evaluation** reviews the effects at the end of the promotion, and may use pre- and post-questioning. It is easy to undertake, involves participants and provides immediate results. **Outcome evaluation** assesses longer-term effects, after collection and analysis of data. It measures sustained changes and provides credibility of data.

2 **Qualitative data** is not statistically based and refers to participant observation and interviews giving a descriptive view. **Quantitative data** measures numerically.

3 When designing a questionnaire the following stages should be gone through: Identify what information you require and from whom. How is the information to be collected – completed by the participant on their own or by interview? How many people in the sample? When will the survey take place? Does the questionnaire need pilot testing? How will the data be analysed and reported?

4 This will include: an overall summary of the research undertaken prior to the activity which supported the need for a health promotion; the methods by which the promotion was delivered and the evaluation of the process and outcomes; conclusions from the analysis of the findings and well-argued recommendations for the future; acknowledgement of individuals and organisations who have given support.

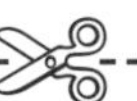

These questions guide you through the topic. If you need help to answer them, look at pages 92–97 of the Collins textbook.

8.9 short **questions** and **activities**

1. Why is it important to undertake an evaluation of a health promotion activity, and what might it show?
2. What are the disadvantages of undertaking evaluation during the process of health promotion?
3. When is an impact evaluation undertaken and what are its advantages?
4. Explain the terms 'reliability' and 'validity' when applied to data collection.
5. Write down the six main considerations before designing a questionnaire.
6. Give an example of an open and a closed question, and describe when it might be appropriate to use each type.
7. What problems are there if the sample size is too small?
8. Describe how the findings from evaluations can be presented.
9. When can conclusions be drawn and what should they be based on?

summaryworksheet

QUESTIONNAIRE DESIGN

Identify the problems in the design of the questionnaire below. All the questions have been worded inappropriately. Identify why, and rewrite them so that they could be successfully used in a questionnaire.

Questionnaire

Please fill in this questionnaire.

1. Are you — under 18 / 18–65 / 65 or over?

2. Do you exercise — Very often / Often / Sometimes / Rarely / Never?

3. Do you think the exercise facilities at college are — Superb / Excellent / Great / Good / Fair / Not so great?

4. Is this the best facility you have ever used? — Yes/No

5. Do you agree with the Principal's plan to support the reduction in college usage of the facility? — Yes/No

6. Do you think the British should eat less and exercise more? — Yes/No

7. Are you against a ban on smoking? — Yes/No

8. Do you agree with the majority of students that the college is failing to promote health? — Yes/No

9. If you were Principal, what would you do to promote health?

10. Is your weight appropriate for your height?

extension**activity**sheet

TYPES OF EVALUATION

Complete this table, remembering that:

- Process evaluation notes reactions to the activity.
- Impact evaluation reviews the effects at the end of the promotion.
- Outcome evaluation assesses longer-term effects.

Activity	*Type of evaluation*	*Ease of undertaking evaluation*	*Comment on accuracy and use of results*
Rates of falls amongst the elderly after a 3-month falls-reduction campaign			
Review of healthy food options in college canteen, 3 months after the introduction of a 'healthy eating' policy			
Take-up levels of a flu immunisation programme			
Questionnaires testing knowledge before and after a health education lesson in school			
Number of leaflets handed out during a health promotion			
Study of no-smoking policies in local restaurants			

Investigating Disease is a portfolio-tested unit and will require students to carry out an investigation into various aspects of two specific diseases, one communicable (viral or bacterial) and one non-communicable. Students will have to show they know about the biological basis of each disease and how the body responds to them. They will need to include information about how the disease is caused and its distribution. They should analyse the availability of support, facilities for diagnosis and treatment in their locality, including the factors that may affect the availability and outcome of the treatments. There should also be an evaluation of the strategies for the prevention of the diseases and the factors that might affect them. To achieve highly with their portfolios, students will need to produce a clear, detailed and in-depth comparison of their two chosen diseases. They should use as wide a range of resources as possible and organise it appropriately and in an effective manner. They should demonstrate a high degree of independence in their work. Whatever level a student is working at, they should follow the specific help given in the assessment guidance section of the specification.

Unit 9

Investigating Disease

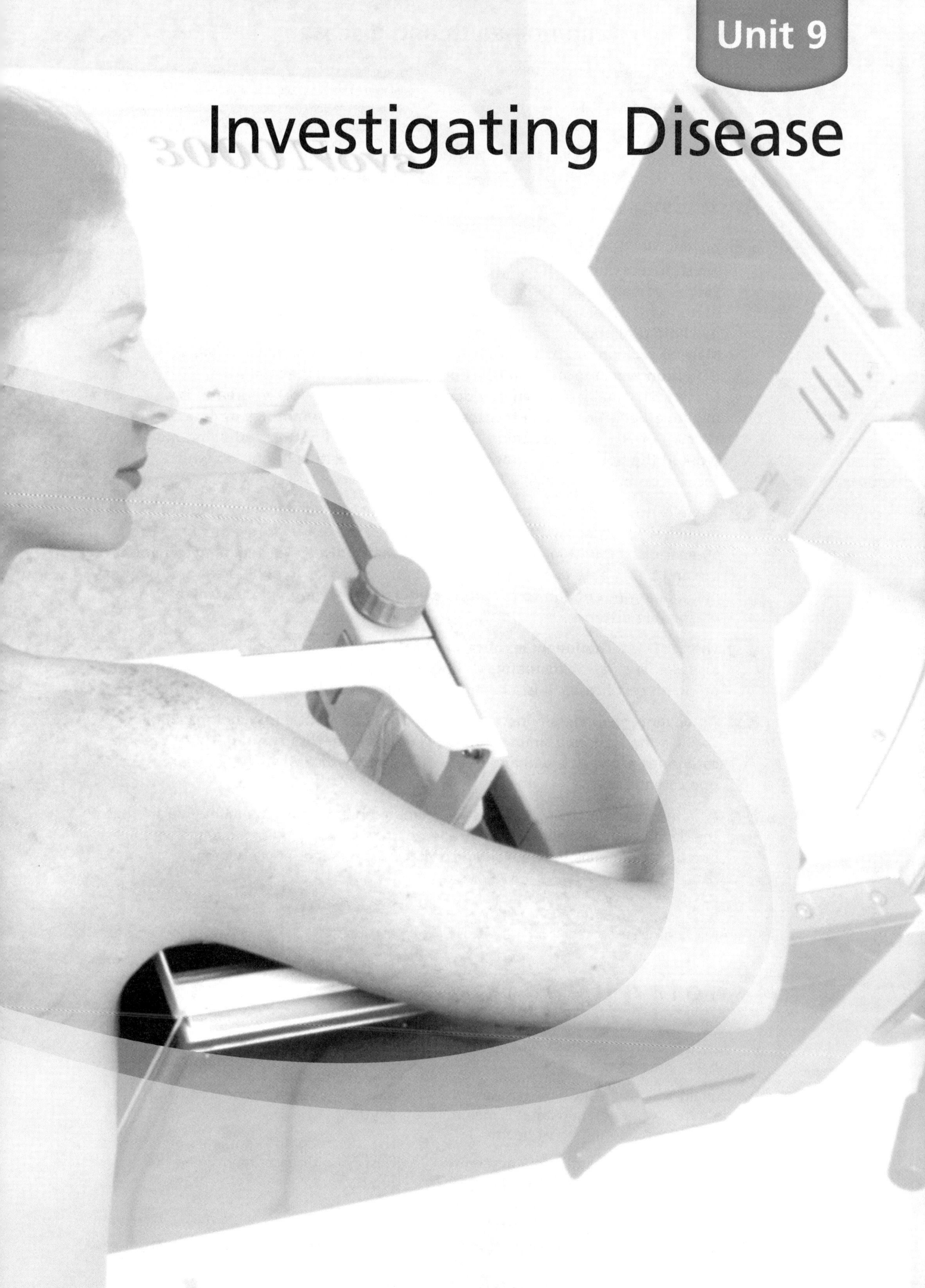

9.1 Understanding health and disease

It is easy to assume that someone studying health and disease should know precisely the meaning of 'health' and 'disease'. These are not easy terms to define. Indeed, there are many definitions. This is one of the main messages in this topic.

Getting you thinking is designed to show that 'being healthy' can mean different things to different people. The pictures should stimulate a discussion and may show there is disagreement about who is most healthy. The students are also encouraged to reflect on times when they were not feeling well. This should introduce them to a range of diseases and what it feels like to be unwell.

Answers to the *Check your understanding* questions on page 105 of the Collins textbook.

1 **Man of 19: 'Health is when you don't have a cold' is a negative definition which focuses on not having a disease or disability.**
Single woman of 20: 'Generally, it's being carefree, you look better, you get on better with other people' is a positive definition which focuses on psychological and social well-being.
Married woman of 28: 'Health is having loads of whumph' is a positive definition which focuses on psychological and social well-being.
Man of 51: 'Health is when you don't feel tired and short of breath' is a negative definition which focuses on being free of symptoms of illness.
Woman of 70: 'Health is being able to walk around better, and doing more work in the house if my knees will let me' is a positive definition which focuses on being physically fit.

2 **There is no one correct answer here. Being healthy to a 20-year-old might mean being physically fit enough to take part in various forms of sport. To a 50-year-old it might mean being free of a major disease or feeling good about life and being able to take part in moderate exercise. To an 80-year-old it might mean being fit enough to carry out daily tasks or being able to walk a reasonable distance.**

3 **The WHO International Classification of Disease is used by those recording diseases, such as epidemiologists and doctors. It is used in hospital records and on death certificates. It is a common 'language' understood in all countries.**

4 **An advantage of classifying diseases as physical, mental (psychological) or social is that it uses a simple or basic classification. Disadvantages are that the categories are very broad and vague. Also, many diseases fall into more than one category.**

5 **Advantages of classifying diseases as communicable and non-communicable are that the classification is simple and fairly easy to understand, and not many diseases fall into both categories. A disadvantage is that the categories are very broad.**

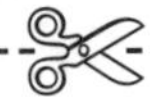

These questions guide you through the topic. If you need help to answer them, look at pages 100–105 of the Collins textbook.

9.1 short **questions** and **activities**

1. Why is it difficult to know what 'health' means?
2. Explain what is meant by a 'negative' definition of health and what is meant by a 'positive' definition of health.
3. Remind yourself what the four different areas of development (PIES) are, and for each area write a sentence that begins, 'Health applies to this area because …'.
4. Why is 'disease' difficult to define?
5. What is the basis for classifying diseases (or indeed, for classifying anything)?
6. List the three different ways of classifying diseases mentioned in this topic.

summary worksheet

COMMUNICABLE OR NON-COMMUNICABLE?

a What do all communicable diseases have in common, in terms of how they are caused?

....

....

b Complete the table by placing a tick in the correct column against each disease.

Name of disease	*Communicable*	*Non-communicable*
Influenza		
Whooping cough		
Heart disease		
Cholera		
Breast cancer		
Athlete's foot		
Multiple sclerosis		
Diabetes		
Pneumonia		
Thrush		
Arthritis		
Down syndrome		
Cystic fibrosis		
Meningitis		

c Choose one communicable disease and one non-communicable disease. Write a short list of some of the differences between the two diseases, e.g. what causes each, which part(s) of the body are affected, and how. You might find this easier if you work with a partner.

HEALTHY OR NOT HEALTHY?

Read this case study and answer the questions that follow.

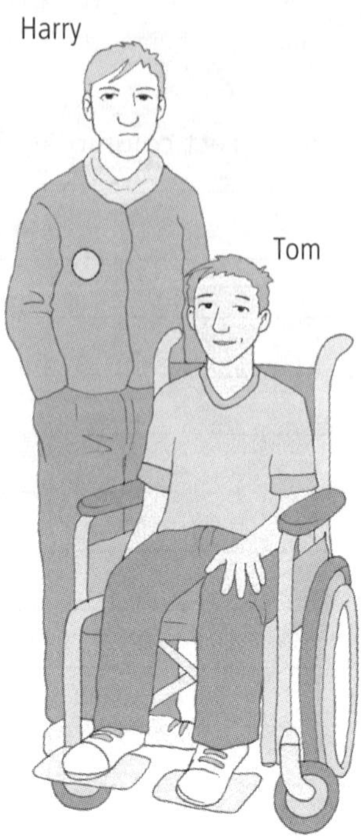

Tom was in a car accident last year and cannot walk at present. The doctors are unsure if he will ever walk again, but Tom is optimistic that he may do. He visits the physiotherapist every week and carries out the exercises that the physiotherapist tells him to do. Tom's family are very supportive and he has many friends who spend a lot of time with him.

Harry is physically very fit. He plays a lot of football but is unpopular. He never passes the ball to anyone as he wants to score all the goals himself. Harry is bad-tempered and he argues with his family a lot. He says that no one understands him.

a Explain who is physically fitter, Tom or Harry?

b Discuss the statement, 'Tom is more healthy that Harry.'

9.2 Exploring epidemiology

This topic introduces epidemiology and looks at its importance in helping an individual who is ill. It is sometimes difficult to see the connection between studying a disease at a population level and how this will impact on individuals. There are many terms which the students may not have met before, such as morbidity or prevalence. These are introduced, along with examples, to make their meaning clear. The historical case study about cholera helps to see 'epidemiology' in action.

Getting you thinking helps focus the students on individuals and populations. It should give a range of possible ways in which information about large groups of people may be gathered. It is important to think about the validity of measurements and why it is important to consider different groups of people.

Answers to the *Check your understanding* questions on page 111 of the Collins textbook.

1 **Epidemiology may be defined as the study of all factors which affect disease in human populations, such as the spread of disease, and the causes of death and disability. It provides valuable information that helps manage an individual person's ill-health.**

2 **The three main areas are: who gets ill?, why do they get ill? and how should they be treated?**

3 **A population pyramid shows a 'snapshot' of a nation's population on a particular day. It shows the number of people, male and female of each age.**

4 **Morbidity statistics show the number of cases of a specified disease occurring in a population at a particular time. They are compiled from hospital records, GPs or disease registers. They are useful for identifying and monitoring trends and so that a quick response to outbreaks of diseases may be made.**

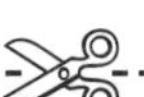

These questions guide you through the topic. If you need help to answer them, look at pages 106–111 of the Collins textbook.

9.2 short questions and activities

1. Explain why studying large groups of people often provides valuable information that helps manage an individual person's ill-health.
2. What is the difference between mortality and morbidity?
3. Explain the importance of aetiology and demography when studying diseases.
4. Give an advantage and a disadvantage of collecting data through a census.
5. Using the information presented in Figure 8, describe how mortality rates for different diseases vary with age.
6. Name five diseases that are 'notifiable'. Find out how many people in your class have had a disease that is notifiable.

summary worksheet

AN EPIDEMIOLOGICAL STUDY – PLAYING AROUND WITH NUMBERS

This table shows the morbidity statistics for some diseases – the numbers of people per 1,000 who contracted the disease.

	Total	20–29 years old	30–39 years old	40–49 years old	50–59 years old	60–69 years old	70+ years old
Stomach cancer	0.66	-	0.25	0.33	0.86	4.23	3.90
Diabetes	16.10	1.67	4.69	23.02	46.59	79.75	49.76
High blood pressure	26.73	2.22	9.38	34.69	82.83	112.91	101.46
Strokes	5.73	0.28	0.25	3.34	12.51	31.05	43.90
Heart disease	11.55	2.22	5.43	16.68	30.20	39.52	44.88
Liver disease	11.95	13.89	13.58	18.01	21.57	23.99	8.78

Source: Korea Institute for Health and Social Affairs, *National Health and Attitude Survey*, 1995

a Which disease was contracted by the highest total number of people?

....

b Which disease was contracted by the lowest total number of people?

....

c Which disease decreased in morbidity for 30–39 year olds compared to 20–29 year olds?

....

d Which disease had the highest morbidity for 20–29 year olds?

....

e Describe how the morbidity of high blood pressure varies with age.

....

....

9.2 extension**activity**sheet

INTERPRETING DATA

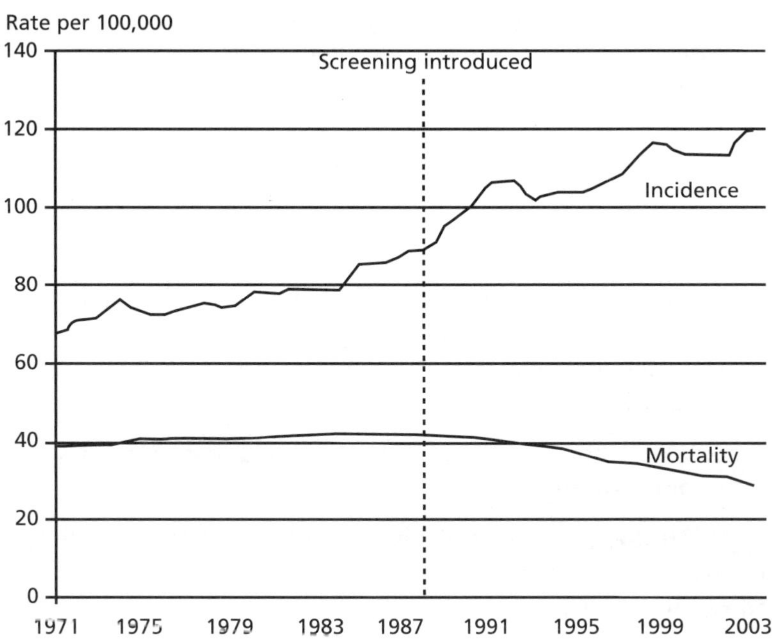

Age-standardised incidence of and mortality from female breast cancer, England, 1971–2003 www.statistics.gov.uk

a Summarise in a short sentence the main message given in the graph.

b Give definitions for incidence and mortality.

c Explain the effect of screening on the incidence and mortality of the breast cancer.

d Find out the importance of presenting the data as age-standardised.

9.3 Communicable diseases

This is a fairly factual topic that looks at the different types of micro-organisms and some of the diseases they cause. It gives information about the structure of the micro-organisms. This helps students to understand how they can affect the body. Knowing about the variety of micro-organisms and diseases will help students make an informed choice about which one they want to study in detail for their portfolio. Some diseases will be familiar and some will be new.

Getting you thinking helps students to focus on illnesses and how they are transmitted by getting them to think about their own experiences. It also gets them thinking about how the transmission of diseases may be reduced. There are sometimes misconceptions about how diseases are spread. It should be emphasised that, rather than the diseases themselves, it is the organisms that cause diseases that are passed from one person to another.

Answers to the *Check your understanding* questions on page 117 of the Collins textbook.

1. **Communicable diseases are caused by micro-organisms. They are 'caught' from other people and can affect us during any life stage. We usually recover from communicable diseases quickly, although this may depend on how old we are and how fit we are.**
2. **Virus, e.g. influenza. Bacterium, e.g. tuberculosis. Fungus, e.g. Athlete's foot. Protozoon, e.g. plasmodium.**
3. **Viruses are smaller than bacteria. Viruses have a simple structure – mainly genetic material surrounded by a protein coat, whereas bacteria have a more complicated cellular structure.**
4. **Air-borne, e.g. influenza. Water-borne, e.g. cholera. Food-borne, e.g. Salmonella food poisoning. Direct-contact, e.g. chickenpox. Through vectors, e.g. malaria.**

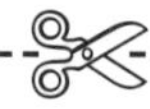

These questions guide you through the topic. If you need help to answer them, look at pages 112–117 of the Collins textbook.

9.3 short **questions** and **activities**

1. Some micro-organisms are 'friendly', whilst others cause diseases. Name two 'friendly' organisms. Which type of organism always causes a disease?
2. Name three bacteria that cause food poisoning.
3. Make a table that shows three systems in the body and some of the diseases that affect them.
4. Describe the two different types of fungal structure. Name a disease caused by a fungus with each type of structure.
5. Explain which is the vector – plasmodium, malaria or mosquito.
6. Explain why the very young and the very old are more susceptible to having diseases such as influenza.

9.3

summaryworksheet

COMMUNICATING ABOUT COMMUNICABLE DISEASES

a Complete the table to show various communicable diseases, the type and the name of the micro-organism that causes them, and their methods of transmission.

Name of disease	*Type of micro-organism causing the disease*	*Name of micro-organism causing the disease*	*Method of transmission*
influenza		Influenza virus	droplet infection
cholera	bacterium	*Vibrio cholera*	
	bacterium	*Staphylococcus aureus*	
Athlete's foot		*Tinea*	
warts	virus		direct contact
		Measles virus	
AIDS	virus		
	protozoon	*Plasmodium*	
		Herpes simplex virus	
whooping cough			
		Escherichia colix	food-borne

b Read the 'Does age matter?' section on page 117. Explain why some people get diseases, whereas others may not, even if disease-causing organisms get inside their bodies.

COMPARING AND CONTRASTING MICRO-ORGANISMS

Here is a diagram of a virus, a bacterium and a fungus.

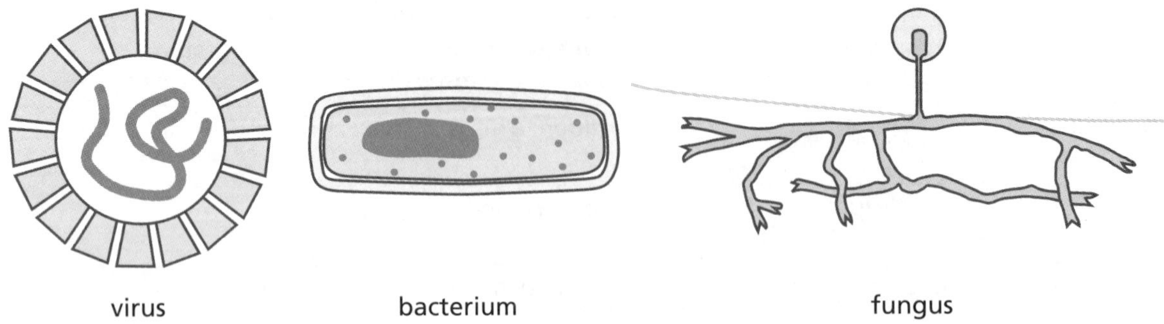

a Make up a table that shows the similarities and differences between viruses, bacteria and fungi. Use the following headings:

- structure of the micro-organism
- diseases caused
- possible mode of entry into the body.

b Find out more about vectors of disease. Write a short paragraph, naming the vectors and the disease-causing organisms they carry. Say how you think the diseases they carry might be eradicated.

9.4 Non-communicable diseases

This topic looks at non-communicable diseases – ones that are not caused by micro-organisms. It is important that the students fully understand the difference between communicable and non-communicable diseases, as they will have to choose one of each to study and compare for their portfolio. Again, like the previous one, this is a factual topic and will help the students to make a choice. It groups the diseases into different categories, giving key up-to-date information about many of the common non-communicable diseases.

Getting you thinking will show that it is not always possible to tell if someone has a disease. Even when it is obvious that someone has an impairment, it is difficult to say how that impairment might have occurred. Students should be encouraged to think about the range of diseases occurring in different age groups.

Answers to the *Check your understanding* questions on page 125 of the Collins textbook.

1 **Non-communicable diseases are not caused by micro-organisms and cannot be 'caught' from another person. They are often associated with lifestyle or the environment. Specific non-communicable diseases tend to affect us during a particular life stage and they usually require long-term treatment and support.**

2 **Degenerative diseases include arthritis, multiple sclerosis, dementia, Parkinson's and cataracts. Each of these diseases tends to get progressively worse as time goes on.**

3 **The two main types of genetic diseases are those that affect whole chromosomes and those that affect single genes. Chromosome defects may affect the number of chromosomes or the order of genes on the chromosomes, whereas defects of single genes involve the order of the DNA bases.**

4 **Atheroma are fatty plaques that build up inside the inner lining of arteries, making the surface rough and the space inside the arteries narrowed. This may stimulate blood-clot formation as the body thinks it needs to repair itself. If this happens in a coronary artery, the blood clot may block or severely restrict the flow of blood carrying food and oxygen to the heart muscle. The muscle cells may die or not be able to contract the heart properly, and this may result in a heart attack.**

5 **A benign tumour is a discrete lump of cells that is harmless, whereas a malignant tumour is a lump of cells that can travel round the body and grow in various organs. A malignant tumour is referred to as cancer.**

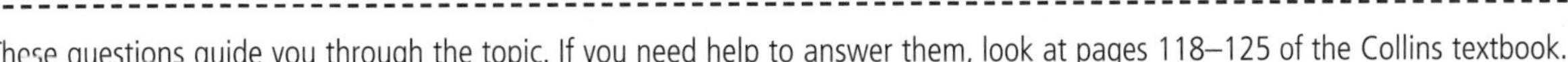

These questions guide you through the topic. If you need help to answer them, look at pages 118–125 of the Collins textbook.

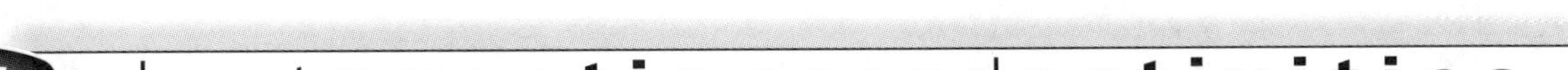

9.4 short questions and activities

1 Make up a table to show the four main categories of non-communicable diseases, their key features and an example of a disease in each category.

2 Name the two types of arthritis.

3 Explain why the diagnosis of Alzheimer's disease is difficult.

4 Name two vitamins and the diseases that occur if there is a lack of them.

5 List as many genetic diseases as you can.

6 Explain why someone with emphysema would not be able to walk far.

7 List the four most common cancers and say why you think most cancers occur when we get older.

summary worksheet

CLASSIFYING NON-COMMUNICABLE DISEASES

a Complete the table by placing a tick in the appropriate box alongside each disease. Note that, for some diseases, you may wish to put a tick in more than one box.

Name of disease	*Degenerative*	*Deficiency*	*Inherited*	*Associated with lifestyle or the environment*
Parkinson's				
Heart disease				
Diabetes				
Cystic fibrosis				
Cataract				
Sickle-cell anaemia				
Alzheimer's				
Emphysema				
Osteoarthritis				
Multiple sclerosis				
Lung cancer				
Down syndrome				
Turner's syndrome				
Stroke				

b Choose a disease where you have put a tick in two boxes. Explain why this disease may be in more than one category.

DIFFERENT FORMS OF ARTHRITIS AND DIABETES

Some diseases have more than one form – arthritis and diabetes, for example. For each of these diseases, summarise the similarities and differences of the two forms of diseases. Present the information in the form of a poster, Powerpoint slides, or a booklet. Use illustrations and tables to make the information as clear as possible to other people.

You may wish to do further research about the different forms of each disease.

9.5 Diagnosis of disease

This topic looks at a variety of methods in which diseases may be diagnosed. It starts off by looking at the clinical features of diseases and distinguishes between signs and symptoms. The importance of early diagnosis is stressed. It is likely that students may well have heard of many of the diagnostic techniques. There are descriptions of how the techniques are used and also the rationale behind them. Different techniques are compared, with advantages and disadvantages highlighted. Students will learn that some techniques are particularly suitable for certain diseases and also that some diseases may be diagnosed using a variety of techniques.

The *Getting you thinking* picture will immediately focus students on signs of a disease. It should be stressed that knowing someone is ill is not always as obvious as this. They may have symptoms that we cannot see. Sometimes symptoms may be vague, and more sophisticated diagnostic techniques need to be employed.

Answers to the *Check your understanding* questions on page 131 of the Collins textbook.

1 **A sign is something that can be seen or measured by someone else, such as spots or a high temperature. A symptom is something that can be felt by someone, but not necessarily be seen by someone else, such as a headache or pain in general.**

2 **It is usually easier to treat a disease if it is diagnosed early. The effect on the body will not be as great and therefore treatment is more likely to be effective, with the person recovering more quickly.**

3 **X-rays are used to detect broken bones or problems with the digestive system if used with a compound such as a barium meal. CAT scans are used to detect problems with soft tissues, such as brain tumours. Nuclear imaging involves using a gamma camera and radionuclides to detect cancers. PET scanning can detect brain tumours, lung cancer and heart disorders. MRI uses magnetism to detect tumours in various body tissues. Ultrasound uses high-frequency sound to detect problems with soft tissues, such as a 'hole' in the heart or abnormal blood flow. Fibre-optic endoscopy is useful for detecting problems with the digestive system.**

4 **Amniocentesis samples the amniotic fluid surrounding the foetus. Chorionic villus sampling samples material from the chorion (developing placenta). The latter technique gives an earlier result, but carries a higher risk of miscarriage.**

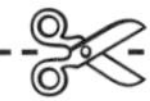

These questions guide you through the topic. If you need help to answer them, look at pages 126–131 of the Collins textbook.

9.5 short **questions** and **activities**

1 What is meant by the clinical features of a disease?

2 Explain why the early detection of a communicable disease is important in reducing its transmission.

3 Explain the difference between an invasive and a non-invasive technique for detecting a disease.

4 In which two body fluids is diabetes normally detected?

5 Explain, in your own words, why bones show up 'light' in X-rays.

6 Define the term 'mammography'.

summary worksheet

WHICH TYPE OF DIAGNOSIS?

The table below gives some clinical features of diseases. Complete the table to show which detection technique would be most suitable, and explain your answer in each case.

Remember that the main detection techniques are:

- Biochemical tests
- Imaging techniques
- Genetic techniques.

Clinical feature of a disease	*Suitable detection technique*	*Explanation of choice of detection technique*
A boy with severe pain in the leg after falling off a bike.		
A baby with an abnormal heart beat, looking 'blue'.		
A man with some bleeding from the rectum.		
A woman who has just discovered a lump in her breast.		
A middle-aged man always feeling thirsty, with a family history of diabetes.		
A 40 year-old woman, pregnant for the first time, having a slight loss of blood.		

DIAGNOSING DISEASES IN DIFFERENT WAYS

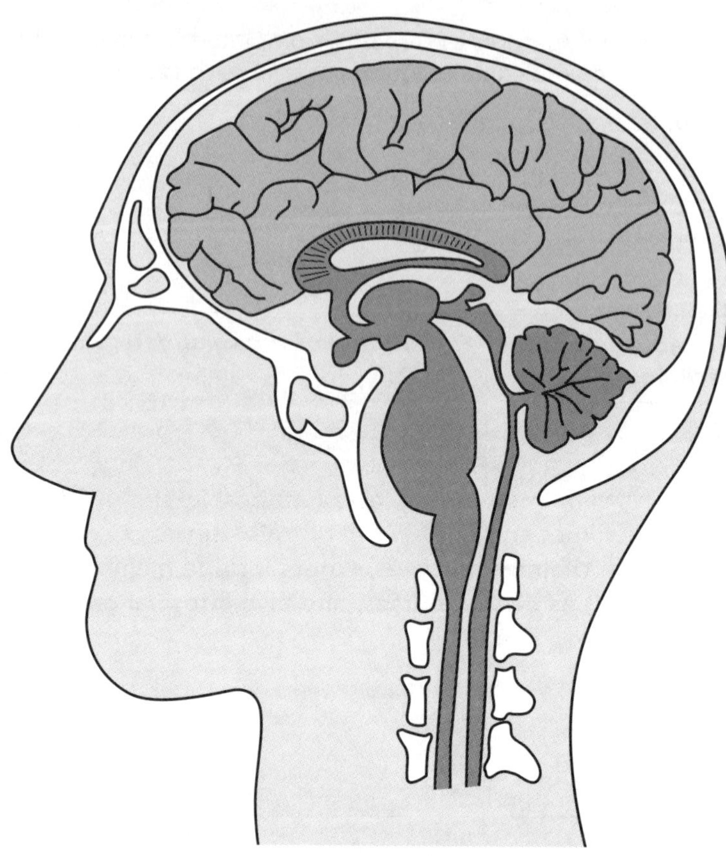

The drawing shows a section through a head, to show the brain and part of the spinal cord. There are different ways of 'seeing' our brains.

a Make a list of the different imaging techniques that allow us to detect problems inside the skull, such as brain tumours.

b Imagine that you are a doctor who has a patient with a suspected brain tumour.

- **i** Explain to the patient as clearly as you can what a brain tumour is.
- **ii** Write out a short paragraph describing the possible techniques that are available for diagnosing brain tumours.
- **iii** For each method, give an advantage and a disadvantage.

9.6 Treatment of disease

This topic shows that diseases may be treated by different people in different places. Examples of such diseases are given. Students may be familiar with their local health centre, and some may well have been in hospital or had serious diseases. Sensitivity should be employed when discussing such issues.

The *Getting you thinking* questions are designed to get students to consider the severity of different diseases and where they should be treated. These are just examples and many more could be discussed. Students may well have some misconceptions, but many will rely on their own personal experience or that of someone in their own family.

Answers to the *Check your understanding* questions on page 137 of the Collins textbook.

1 **Diseases such as Athlete's foot or headaches may be treated by individuals themselves. High blood pressure or bacterial infection such as a sore throat are usually treated in a local practice. Operations to set a broken leg or removal of an appendix are carried out in a local hospital. Specialist, national centres or hospitals would treat people with cancer or heart disease or eye problems.**

2 **Charities and support groups include the British Heart Foundation which supports people with heart disease, or Epilepsy Research Foundation which supports people with epilepsy. Clinics, often at local health practices, include high blood pressure clinics and diabetes clinics. Domestic care refers to the care that people receive in their own homes. Carers include members of the Primary Health Care team, such as district nurses, and also informal carers, such as relatives and neighbours.**

3 **The main factors that can affect the availability of support and treatment regimes for a disease include self-diagnosis and treatment, cost of medicines and other consumables, availability of specialist staff and the need for specialist equipment. Someone with breast cancer may not seek help soon enough after discovering a lump. They may have to wait some time before being treated due to a shortage of specialist staff and the availablity of specialist equipment. Someone with influenza may find it expensive to buy medicines (not through prescription). They may have needed a vaccine, but there may have not been enough available in their area.**

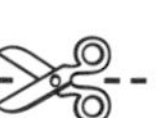

These questions guide you through the topic. If you need help to answer them, look at pages 132–137 of the Collins textbook.

9.6 short **questions** and **activities**

1 Look at the list of reasons why people choose to treat themselves. Put the items in the order you think is most common. Discuss your results with a partner.

2 Make a list of people who are primary health care staff.

3 What is the most common reason people are prescribed drugs?

4 Who or what is treated at an Outpatients Department?

5 Describe the type of support given by an organisation such as the National Meningitis Trust.

6 Which groups of people are exempt from paying prescriptions charges?

7 List as many pieces of specialist equipment found in a hospital as you can. Compare your list with someone else's.

9.6

summary worksheet

WHICH DEPARTMENT SHOULD I VISIT?

CHAPEL
MATERNITY
MALE WARD
FEMALE WARD
UROLOGY
CONCOURSE
CARDIOLOGY
A & E
X-RAY DEPARTMENT
TOILETS

Finding your way round a hospital, whether as a patient or a visitor can be daunting. Complete this table to show which department to visit or which disease you are having treatment for.

Department to visit	*Disease being treated*
Cardiology	
Podiatry	
	Mental illness
	Skin complaint
Urology	
	A broken ankle
	Rheumatoid arthritis
Radiology	
	Alzheimer's
Oncology	
	Removal of a wisdom tooth

DOMESTIC CARE

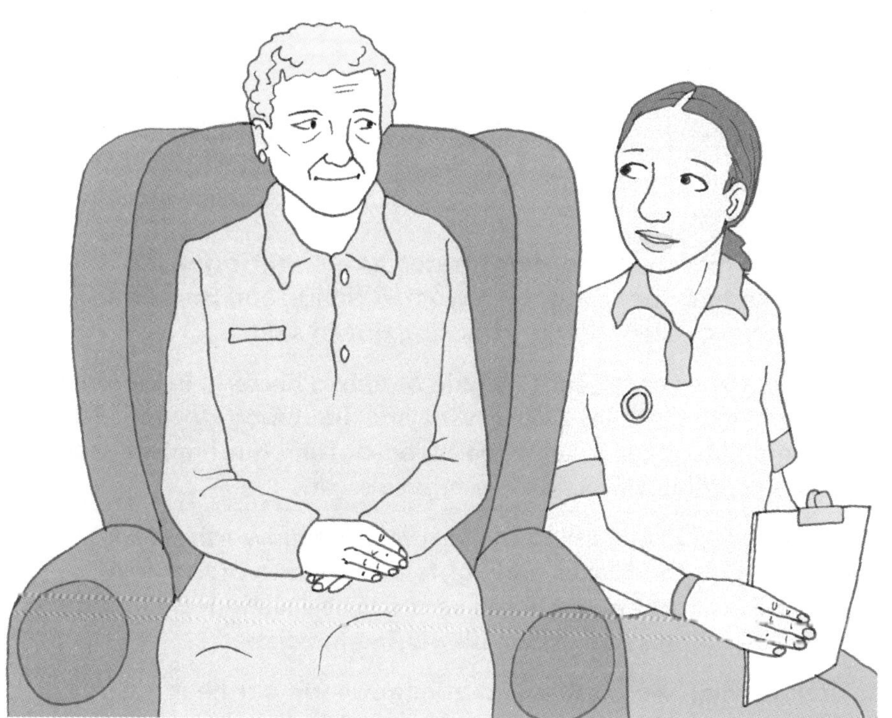

The drawing shows an elderly lady having a visit from a young care worker.

a Suggest a list of tasks that might be undertaken by a care worker when visiting an elderly person.

b Define the term 'informal care worker' and give examples of such people.

c Discuss the statement, 'Elderly people should not need formal care if they have families of their own'.

9.7 Disease-prevention strategies

This topic looks at ways in which we can help prevent ourselves getting ill. This is not always possible, but we can reduce our chances. It starts by looking at the natural defences our bodies have and our immune system. This leads on to national strategies, which include the National Health Service immunisation schedule. There are also many strategies at a local level and our own personal lifestyle choices. Students should be encouraged to examine other examples of strategies in these categories and to consider their impact.

The *Getting you thinking* picture is 'shocking'. It is designed to be, and comes from a real 'anti-smoking' campaign. The students are asked to consider its impact. They should do this in as much depth as they can. There will be much debate why some people continue to smoke.

Answers to the *Check your understanding* questions on page 143 of the Collins textbook.

1 **The three levels of disease-prevention strategies are: national, e.g. the NHS immunisation schedule; local, e.g. well-women clinics; and personal lifestyle choices, e.g. exercising or choosing not to smoke.**

2 **The body's natural lines of defence include harmless bacteria living on or inside the body, skin, epithelial tissue, lysozyme and blood clotting. People who are haemophiliacs have a defective blood-clotting mechanism. Our skin no longer offers as good protection if we have a cut.**

3 **An MOT is a basic check on a car to make sure it is roadworthy. Part of it includes checking that the brakes and lights are working properly. At a well-women clinic, checks are made to see if our basic health is OK. Checks include weight, blood pressure and testing urine for diabetes.**

4 **Risk behaviour is when we do things that might harm our health. Such behaviour includes smoking, excessive alcohol, illicit drug use, unprotected sex and excess dieting.**

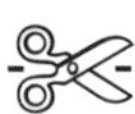

These questions guide you through the topic. If you need help to answer them, look at pages 138–143 of the Collins textbook.

9.7 short **questions** and **activities**

1. Explain how using a handkerchief is a good example of a disease-prevention strategy.
2. Draw a flow chart to show how our immune system deals with a pathogen that has entered our body.
3. Name two infectious diseases that have been a 'global' concern in recent years.
4. Explain the benefits of having health information booklets available in medical practices.
5. Design a poster, aimed at young children, explaining the importance of personal hygiene.
6. Write a paragraph summarising the information given in Figure 39 about drug misuse.

summary worksheet

WHICH TYPE OF STRATEGY?

a Which type of strategy is each of these disease-prevention measures? Tick the correct box.

Disease-prevention measure	*Personal strategy*	*Local strategy*	*National strategy*
Washing hands before preparing food			
A night-class in yoga in a secondary school			
A well-men clinic in a health centre			
Going for a 2-mile run every morning			
Attending a swimming class			
A smoking ban in all places where food is served			
Making a New Year resolution to stop smoking			
A 4-mile run organised by a city council			
Advertising 'Eat five portions of fruit and veg each day'			

b Give *one* advantage of national disease-prevention strategies over local disease-prevention strategies.

....

....

c Give *one* advantage of local disease-prevention strategies over national disease-prevention strategies.

....

....

extension**activity**sheet

HOW REALISTIC ARE NATIONAL AIMS?

The National Heart Forum's policy goals for the prevention of heart disease

- A national coordinated and sustained strategy is needed to increase fruit and vegetable consumption to help people achieve the goal of at least five portions of fruit and vegetables a day.
- Schools and local authorities should support a whole-school approach to food, which promotes consistent healthy eating messages in the school dining room, in tuck shops and vending machines and in the classroom.
- Nutritional standards for school meals should be carefully monitored to ensure that meals meet established quantified nutritional recommendations, and the standards should be strengthened as necessary.
- Emphasis should be placed on school nutrition-education programmes, including practical food skills for all children, such as cooking and meal planning.
- In addition to the Department of Health, the Food Standards Agency should contribute to the formulation of a national nutrition policy, as well as dealing with food safety issues.
- Neighbourhood renewal strategies should combat food deserts by attracting local shops into deprived areas through planning and business incentives, and promote healthy eating by encouraging discount schemes for the purchase of fruit and vegetables.
- Government should work with the food industry to make healthy changes to processed and pre-prepared foods by reducing levels of fat, sugar and salt.

a Make a table with the headings 'Achieved', 'Partially achieved' and 'Not yet achieved'.

b Place each of the NHF's goals into a category in your table.

c For each goal, explain your choice of category.

d Add one more goal of your choice, and explain which category you would place it in.

9.8 Factors affecting disease prevention

Having considered disease prevention in the previous topic, this topic examines some of the reasons why disease-prevention strategies do not always work. Some people think, 'It will not happen to me'. Others will not agree with what the doctor tells them, or if they do, they may not follow the advice given. Examples of such cases are given. Students should also realise the importance of doctors not over-prescribing antibiotics, and the fact that there is not a bottomless sack of money available for health.

The picture in the *Getting you thinking* section is becoming a familiar sight in some of our towns and cities. It should focus the students on the idea of public perception of risk. Students may well have their own opinions about why people behave like this, even when they know the dangers of what they are doing. They may well come up with their own ideas of who might be able to change such behaviour, and how. The discussion could be widened to include other areas in which the public's perception of risk is not rational.

Answers to the *Check your understanding* questions on page 149 of the Collins textbook.

1 **Some people may have a poor perception of risk, such as young people not knowing the dangers of drinking excessive alcohol. This might result in liver disease later in life. Some patients might not agree with what the doctor tells them. Examples include tranquillisers not being readily accepted, or being prescribed antibiotics. The consequences of these actions might mean that the patient might not get better quickly. Some patients do not always follow the advice given by a doctor. Examples include not finishing a course of medicine or not following a healthy lifestyle. As a consequence, the patient may not recover fully. Antibiotic resistance occurs when too many antibiotics are prescribed. This means that they will no longer be effective, and this could be dangerous if someone contracts a dangerous bacterial disease. The amount of funding affects the prevention of disease. Most people have to pay a contribution to prescriptions, dental treatment and glasses. Some people might not be able to afford this or may not want to pay for dental treatment or checkups.**

2 **People agreed most with being prescribed antibiotics. The effects of antibiotics are well known and most are effective. People agreed least with being prescribed tranquillisers. It is known some tranquillisers are addictive and people could be frightened that they might become dependent on them and take them for longer than necessary.**

3 **Patients sometimes do not comply with doctors' recommendations because they are not satisfied with their consultation, they do not understand the information they were given or they could not remember what they were told.**

4 **There are more antibiotic-resistant bacteria today because of their increased use. Some bacteria may mutate (have a change in their genes) and become resistant. These bacteria are not killed by the antibiotic and go on to reproduce, thus increasing in number. This means that the antibiotic is ineffective against an increasingly large number of bacteria.**

5 **Funding comes from the Treasury which is the central government department responsible for balancing the country's finances. The NHS has to compete with other departments each year for money, and sometimes the government might have a higher priority for other departments, such as education or defence.**

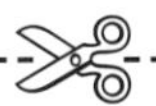

These questions guide you through the topic. If you need help to answer them, look at pages 144–149 of the Collins textbook.

9.8 short **questions** and **activities**

1. List the four reasons given to explain why most people have an unreal perception of risk.
2. Describe two examples in which the media have heightened our awareness of risk.
3. Explain, as clearly and simply as you can, the difference between concordance and compliance.
4. Give six ways in which doctors could help to increase patient compliance.
5. Who was the person responsible for creating the modern welfare state?
6. Make a timeline to show the important events in funding available for health.

DIFFERENT WAYS OF PRESENTING DATA

The table shows the number of antibiotic prescriptions dispensed in England.

Year	*Prescription items (millions)*
1991	43.7
1992	43.4
1993	47.7
1994	45.8
1995	49.4
1996	46.6
1997	46.4
1998	42.6
1999	38.6
2000	36.9

a Plot the data as a bar chart, on the graph paper below.

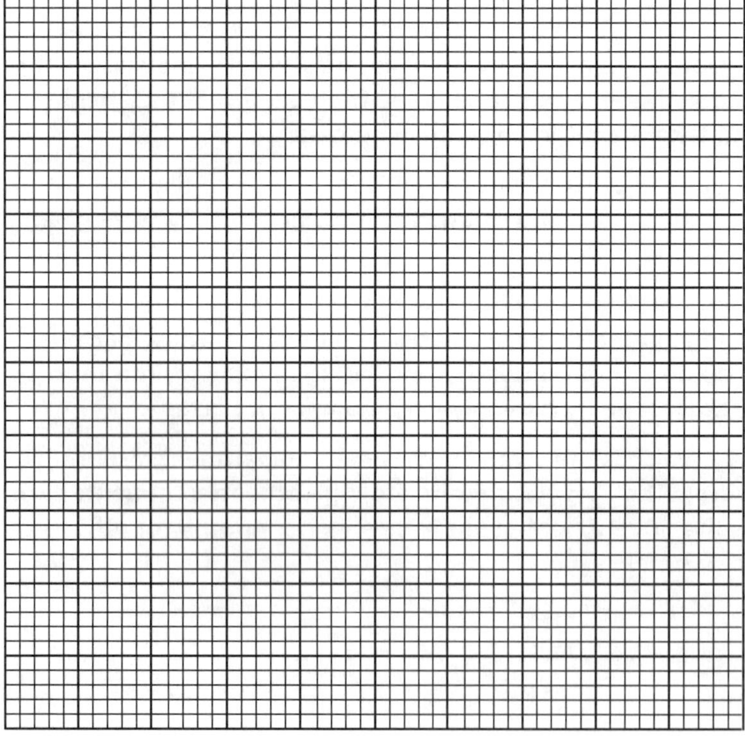

b Describe the trend shown by the graph from 1991 to 2000.

....

....

c Explain whether you think the graph shows the data more clearly than the table.

....

....

....

DOCTOR–PATIENT RELATIONSHIPS

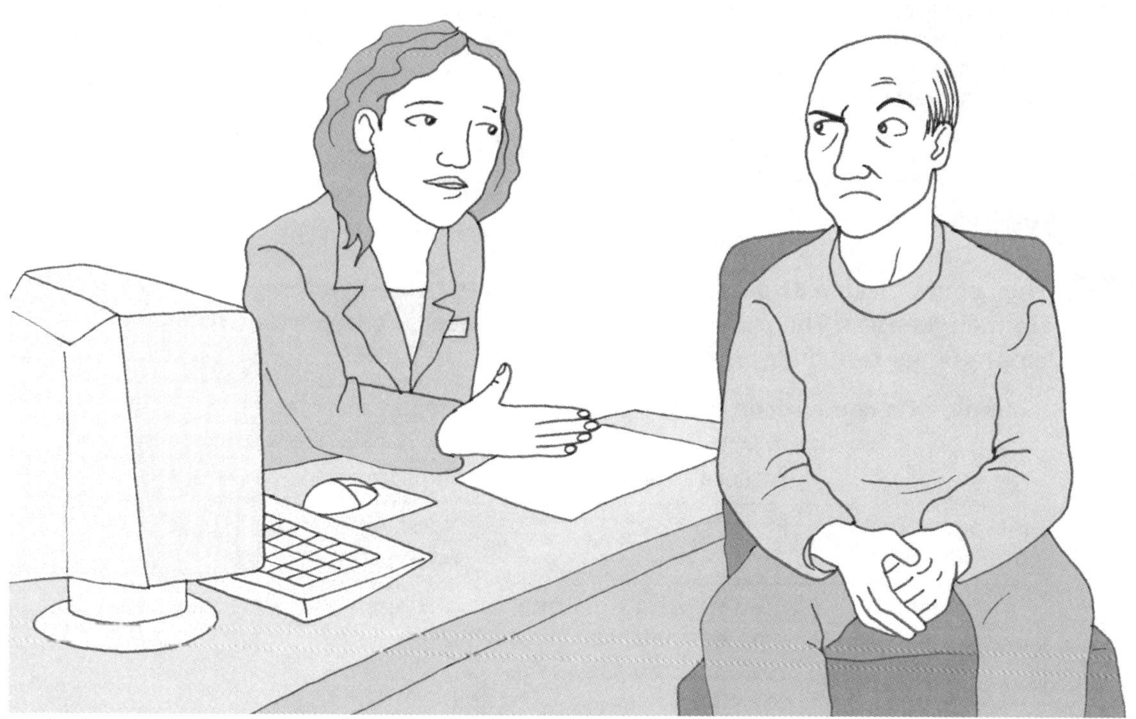

a Re-read the paragraph about 'Patient–doctor concordance' and repetitive strain injury (RSI) on page 145. Write a short paragraph, entitled, 'The doctor always knows best'.

b Imagine you are a doctor and you have a patient who is overweight and has signs of heart disease. You tell the patient that they 'must lose weight and stop smoking'. You then prescribe the patient tablets for high blood pressure.

- **i** Look at the advice given (end of page 146) for ensuring patient compliance. Now re-write what you tell this patient.
- **ii** Now, imagine that you are talking to the patient's partner. What advice would you give to them to ensure patient compliance?
- **iii** Outline the main differences in the advice you would give to the patient and to the patient's partner.

9.9 Putting it all together: case studies

This final topic gathers the ideas from the previous topics and helps the students focus on comparing diseases, an important element of their portfolios. Pairs of diseases are introduced as part of case studies. The case studies are grouped according to where the diagnosis or treatment is being carried out. The students are shown how to use tables for easy summary comparisons, although it should be stressed that more detailed information will be needed for high marks in their portfolios.

Getting you thinking will help focus on different diseases. There should be much discussion about what might be wrong with the people in the picture. The range of people they might be waiting to see will obviously differ depending on what diseases the students come up with. This could also be approached by considering the people they might be waiting to see first and which diseases might be diagnosed or treated by each of these people.

Answers to the *Check your understanding* questions on page 155 of the Collins textbook.

1 **The communicable diseases are food poisoning, Athlete's foot, AIDS and German measles. The non-communicable diseases are hypertension, emphysema, testicular cancer and autism.**

Example of a comparison of two of these diseases in a table:

	Athlete's foot	**Hypertension**
Biological basis of disease	Fungus, *Tinea*	Narrowing of the arteries or a very fast heart beat
Transmission	Contact with someone who has had the disease, such as using the same towel or walking barefoot.	Not applicable, but related to lifestyle
Signs	Flaky or broken skin between the toes	Both systolic and diastolic blood pressure being significantly above normal for age
Symptoms	Itchiness between the toes	Feeling stressed
Further confirmation of diagnosis	Not usually necessary	Angiogram (scan of blood vessels in the brain) to check on how much the blood vessels have narrowed. This will only be done if it is thought that the hypertension is a significant risk to future health.
Treatment	Fungicidal cream	Prescribing medication to reduce blood pressure. Change in lifestyle, to include healthier diet and exercise. Steps taken to help reduce stress.

2

	Meningitis	Heart attack
Biological basis of disease	Meningitis virus or bacterium, e.g. *Neisseria meningitidis*	Build up of atheroma in coronary arteries, leading eventually to severely reduced blood flow to the heart muscle.
Transmission	Contact with someone who has had the disease.	Not applicable, but related to lifestyle
Signs	Similar to flu,such as fever and perhaps vomiting. A rash may be present.	Patient clearly in discomfort, perhaps collapsed.
Symptoms	Similar to flu such as headaches, feeling tired and sick. Also stiff neck.	Crushing chest pain
Diagnosis	Isolation of the virus or bacterium	ECG (electrocardiogram)
Treatment	Antibiotics if bacterial.	Initially, rest in intensive care, blood-thinning drugs. Change in lifestyle.

3 **Food poisoning may be prevented by good hygiene. People preparing food should make sure they wash their hands, keep cooked and non-cooked meat separate, etc. Hypertension may be prevented, to some extent, by adopting a healthy lifestyle such as exercising, eating sensibly and not smoking.**

These questions guide you through the topic. If you need help to answer them, look at pages 150–155 of the Collins textbook.

9.9 short **questions** and **activities**

1. List the seven aspects under which you need to compare your chosen communicable and non-communicable diseases.
2. Make a list of the characteristics of the town in which John, the GP lives.
3. Describe the factors that might affect the diagnosis and treatment of Amir's and Fatima's diseases.
4. From the evidence given, explain how we can tell that emphysema is a more serious disease than Athlete's foot.
5. Explain why Damien's father is reluctant for Damien to be immunised.
6. Explain the role of Nazy, the triage nurse.
7. Read the paragraph about the factors affecting the diagnosis, treatment and prevention of Tom's and Angus's diseases. Compare the information about the two diseases in a table.

summary worksheet

A BUSY ACCIDENT AND EMERGENCY DEPARTMENT

Read the case study and answer the questions that follow.

> Dr Reed is in charge of a busy accident and emergency (A&E) department of a large city hospital. It is a Saturday evening and there are many patients being brought in. One patient is 18-year-old Ted, who has been involved in a road accident and has a serious head wound. Dr Reed attends to Ted immediately. Another patient is 15-year-old Maria, who has suspected food poisoning. She is the sixth patient who has been brought in with similar symptoms today. Five-year-old Reuben is brought in by his parents, because they suspect he has measles. Although Reuben is very young, his parents are told they may have to wait some time to be seen. Other people waiting to be seen are Chei, who thinks he may have broken his arm, and Peter, who is feeling dizzy.

a Some of the diseases are communicable and others are non-communicable.

i List the communicable diseases.

....

....

ii List the non-communicable diseases.

....

....

b Not all the people can be seen immediately.

i Put the people in the order that they should be seen.

....

....

ii Explain your choice of order.

....

....

....

....

extension**activity**sheet

FINDING OUT ABOUT DISEASES

Your task here is to collect information about different diseases from as many people as you can, and then analyse the information. This could be a big task, so you will first have to decide how many different diseases – and which ones – you are going to find out about.

a Make up a questionnaire that you will give out. (Remember, you should treat the information you receive confidentially and that no one should be asked to fill in the questionnaire if they do not want to.) The questionnaire should gather the following information:

- How old the person was when they had the disease
- What signs and symptoms they had
- Whether they visited the doctor
- Whether they had to go to hospital
- What treatment they had.

b Present the information in the form of tables and graphs. Remember to give each a heading so that it is clear to others what the information shows.

c Summarise the conclusions of your findings.

d Compare the primary information you found with that of secondary sources such as books or the internet. If there are any major differences in the information, can these be explained?

Understanding Research in Health and Social Care is a portfolio-tested unit and will require students to carry out a research project in which they obtain and use both primary and secondary data. The research investigation should cover a topic that is relevant to the health and social care field. The topic may be drawn from one or more of the units within the GCE Health and Social Care (Double Award), concerning the following client groups: people who are ill, young children, older people, people with specific needs. The assessment evidence should contain a research proposal and a written report. Students need to make sure that they demonstrate their ability to use basic research skills. They will have to demonstrate knowledge and understanding of research methodology and use relevant techniques to obtain research data. The report should contain analysis of the student's data and an evaluation of the project and the methodology used. To achieve highly with their portfolios, students will need to produce a clear, detailed, structured research proposal. They should demonstrate a high level of knowledge and understanding, both of their topic and of the research methodology. Their report should use correct specialist vocabulary and demonstrate an excellent level of analytical thinking. The students should demonstrate a high degree of independence in their work.

Whatever level a student is working at, they should follow the specific help given in the assessment guidance section of the specification.

Unit 10

Understanding Research in Health and Social Care

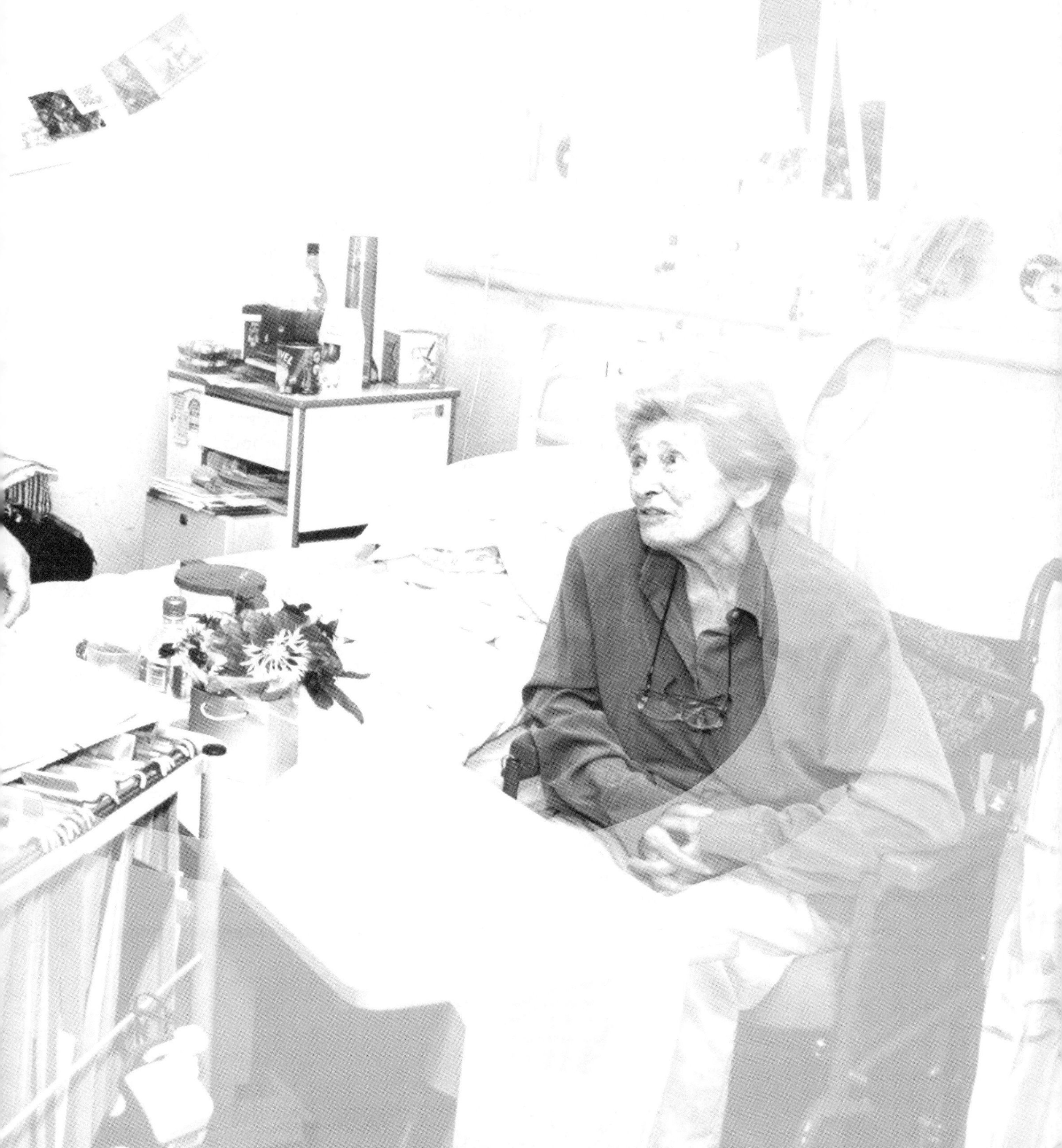

10.1 Introducing health and social care research

The rationale behind this first topic is to help students to understand that scientific research and effective care practice and policy should be inseparable. Research findings offer care professionals and policy-makers cutting-edge knowledge that can be used for the benefit of the community and society. In getting this point across, the teacher might refer, for example, to studies of successful interventions, such as clinical trials and patient satisfaction surveys.

Because Unit 10 offers guidance for students on how to conduct their own, small-scale research project, the teacher is in a position to let students find out by themselves what scientific research can uncover, rather than just trusting the textbook.

In addition to the importance of choosing the right method for the right job, students should be reminded that their first and foremost duty as researchers is not to harm the people they are studying and not to put themselves at risk.

Answers to the *Check your understanding* questions on page 163 of the Collins textbook.

1 **Research-based evidence consists of findings that are based on systematic investigation.**

2 **Research-based evidence can help care professionals to make practice decisions that are supported by the latest and most reliable scientific findings.**

3 **Quantitative data: an example is the percentage of patients who benefit from clinical intervention X, compared to clinical intervention Y. This information can help clinicians to choose the best treatment.**
Qualitative data: an example is the text of an interview that describes people's experiences of poverty in their own words. This information reminds policymakers of the human tears that hide behind 'mundane' statistics, hopefully galvanising a humanitarian as well as an arithmetical response.

4 **By checking their findings with each other, scientists can make decisions that are based on collectively agreed fact rather than on impromptu conjecture.**

5 **Systematic reviews contain the distilled wisdom of many research studies, thereby helping researchers to map the current state of play without having to rediscover it.**

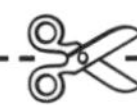

These questions guide you through the topic. If you need help to answer them, look at pages 158–162 of the Collins textbook.

10.1 short **questions** and **activities**

1. Give an example of how an advance in health or social care has depended on the work of researchers.
2. Explain what governance of research means.
3. What is the difference between research evidence and craft knowledge? Need the two be contradictory?
4. Give two examples of objective evidence that relate to research in health and social care.
5. Why should researchers act ethically?
6. Why should researchers investigate existing practice and seek to break new ground?

10.1 **summary**worksheet

KEY TERMS

Look at the definitions of the key terms below. Then provide one (concrete) example of each. To help get you started, we have done the first exercise for you.

a **Research-based evidence**: Findings that are based on data collected through systematic investigation.

An example of research-based evidence is the scientific finding that smoking increases the risk of lung cancer.

b **Evidence-based practice**: Practice that applies the best available evidence, some of it available from research studies, some of it gained from practical experience.

c **Governance of research**: The process of applying and monitoring approved research 'rules' and procedures.

d **Qualitative data**: Non-numerical data – usually presented as 'talk' or 'text', though they can also include images and objects – that provide some form of information.

e **Quantitative data**: Information presented in numerical form. Typically, this involves some form of quantifiable measure.

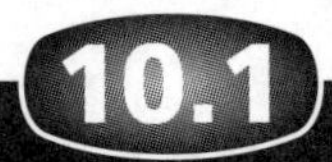

extension**activity**sheet

HOW CAN RESEARCH IMPROVE CARE PRACTICE AND POLICY?

This unit considers how research can produce real health and social benefits for the individual and the community. Consider the following issues and suggest how researchers might be able to contribute to evidence-based practice and policy in health and social care:

a The development of a public health campaign.

b Ensuring that policy and practice address current trends regarding births, morbidity and mortality.

c The most effective way to deal with one of the following disorders: depression; large bowel cancer; obsessive–compulsive disorder; obesity.

d The most effective way to deal with one of the following social problems: poverty; unemployment; long hospital waiting lists; difficulties that disabled people face on public transport.

e How to prevent heart disease.

f How to prevent the development of suicidal tendencies.

10.2 The nature of scientific research

The rationale behind this topic is to foster a better understanding of the application of scientific knowledge. Science allows care researchers to test propositions against hard evidence, which, in turn, leads to the development of objective knowledge. Objectivity is a crucial guard against whim, hearsay and taken-for-granted habits because it forces researchers, practitioners and policy-makers to strive for the best-won argument.

In defence of this position, the students could be pointed to noteworthy advances in health and social care that are anchored in solid and consistent research.

Answers to the *Check your understanding* questions on page 167 of the Collins textbook.

1 This is mainly because health care variables are typically fewer in number but greater in complexity than social care variables. Moreover, many health care researchers are able to use experimental or quasi-experimental designs, which yield very precise data. These designs are harder to replicate in social care research because society is a relatively unwieldy environment compared to the more controllable settings of experimental research. That said, the quasi-experiment does have a place in some social care research.

2 Social care research into how, for example, better wheelchair design can improve mobility and access for disabled people could offer a concrete benefit, provided research findings are acted upon in new design and production.

3 Care research sets out to improve the human condition. It is therefore imperative that care researchers do all that they can to avoid harming those whom they study.

4 This information helps patients, in consultation with their care professionals, to make evidence-based decisions in relation to the most appropriate treatment. Giving the patient an informed voice is not only respectful, it also enables him or her to consider circumstances that could affect treatment choice (e.g. family issues) that clinicians might not be aware of.

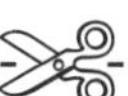

These questions guide you through the topic. If you need help to answer them, look at pages 164–167 of the Collins textbook.

10.2 short **questions** and **activities**

1. Give three examples of empirical evidence.
2. For how long is a scientific claim to be trusted?
3. What is the objection to an 'indifferent social science'?
4. What does it mean to evaluate a care intervention or care policy?
5. Why is it unwise to ignore the scientific evaluation of varying (sometimes competing) care interventions?
6. How can a meta-analysis help health researchers to arrive at the most plausible conclusion?

summary worksheet

SCIENCE

a Identify as many characteristics of science as you can.

b It is probably unwise to suggest that scientific knowledge is entirely factual. Why is this so? As well as using material in the topic to answer the question, refer to other relevant arguments too.

c Identify one example of a 'reliable' care research finding and one example of a 'valid' care research finding, and indicate how the terms 'reliable' and 'valid' apply to each. Make sure you understand what 'reliable' and 'valid' mean first.

d Propose a simple hypothesis about a care issue, and indicate how you might try to test it. An example might be 'More men than women have heart disease.'

10.2 extension**activity**sheet

EVALUATING CARE PRACTICE

The *Evaluating care practice* section (page 166) describes how the scientific evaluation of care practice can help practitioners to discover and replicate good practice, and identify and rectify bad practice.

a Identify one example of good care practice and one example of bad care practice, other than the two examples that are mentioned in the section.

b The section in the textbook describes a meta-analysis of two rival appliances for keeping blood flowing through diseased heart arteries. Imagine that you are a health professional and that you want to explain to a heart patient what a review of the two appliances has shown. Use language that a layperson would understand.

c Using the internet and/or other sources, find another example of a review of two or more care interventions. Write a short, clear summary of your findings in your own words.

10.3 Current practice and new ground

The rationale behind this topic is to help students to understand that change in care practice does not always have to (nor should) start from scratch, whereby a new approach totally replaces a current approach. It is better if effective current practice and the search for even better solutions go hand-on-hand.

In conveying this point, it is worthwhile to consider concrete examples of measures that have 'stood the test of time', those that have been refined and those that have been replaced. It is also important to emphasise the significant role that systematic reviews play in identifying and evaluating best current practice.

Answers to the *Check your understanding* questions on page 171 of the Collins textbook.

1 A systematic review evaluates a number of research studies, whereas an audit evaluates a particular practice or policy against predefined benchmarks.

2 A meta-analysis is a particular kind of systematic review. Its orientation is quantitative. This research instrument is helpful in clinical studies because it puts a figure on the effectiveness of an intervention. For example, a meta-analysis might conclude that 75 per cent of relevant studies indicate that treatment X improved wound healing in burn victims in a range of different hospitals.

3 Three examples are: testing a new medication for heartburn; trying out a range of different exercise regimes for obese patients; and comparing a range of therapies for the treatment of depression. In each case, the proof of the pudding is to be found in the evaluation of different effects. If a new medication for heartburn is found to be better than a current medication, if an innovative exercise regime produces greater and more sustainable weight loss than other regimes, and if a particular therapy significantly enhances patient well-being compared to other therapies, then the clinical trial will have served its purpose. It will have scientifically identified the intervention that will most likely produce the best results.

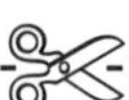

These questions guide you through the topic. If you need help to answer them, look at pages 168–171 of the Collins textbook.

10.3 short **questions** and **activities**

1. How can researchers evaluate existing care measures?
2. How can researchers find better care solutions?
3. How can the identification of poor practice help care practitioners?
4. What ethical issues might arise in offering a promising treatment to one group of patients but not to another group in order to find out if the treatment really works?
5. Why is it difficult to conduct experiments in non-clinical settings?
6. What does it mean to 'enjoy the best of both worlds' with regard to current practice and new ground?

10.3 **summary**worksheet

EXISTING MEASURES AND NEW SOLUTIONS

Complete the table by identifying reasons for evaluating two named existing care measures and reasons for exploring new solutions to two named care problems.

Existing care measure 1:
Reason for evaluating:

Existing care measure 2:
Reason for evaluating:

Care problem 1:
Reason for exploring new solutions:

Care problem 2:
Reason for exploring new solutions:

'STATE OF THE ART' THINKING

Using the internet and other relevant sources, investigate current 'state of the art' thinking on anti-poverty measures in the UK or in a local area. Show your findings to the rest of the class in a short Powerpoint presentation, distinguishing, as appropriate, between existing policies and new proposals.

You might find it useful to work in pairs for this activity.

10.4 Ethics in care research

The rationale behind this topic is to impress upon students the need not only to do care research, but also to care for the people whom they study. In that context, students need to understand that unethical research has caused great human suffering. Nazi experiments are a powerful reminder here. Not only must ethics govern how research is conducted, but how research findings are used as well.

It is also important to consider the issues and application of 'beneficence' and 'distributive justice' when carrying out research, particularly when putting forward evidence-based proposals.

Answers to the *Check your understanding* questions on page 177 of the Collins textbook.

1 **Three examples of ethical research principles are: to protect participants' right to dignity; to involve, whenever appropriate, hard-to-reach groups in the actual research process; to obtain informed consent from participants.**

2 **High ethical standards are vital because care research is not just about finding ways to improve care practice and policy – it must also involve caring for the well-being of participants during the research process.**

3 **There is no easy answer to this question. A small degree of deception (later disclosed to the participant) is arguably permissible if it is vital for the study. For example, the use of a placebo without the participant's prior knowledge might help researchers to determine if an inactive substance is less effective in pain control than an active ingredient. If a degree of deception is proposed, then an independent ethics review board should approve the proposal. Blatant lies and serious underhandedness are always inexcusable.**

4 **'Distributive justice' refers to the fair allocation of resources in society. Ethical social policies aim to ensure that the allocation of public goods and services is based on need rather than ability to pay.**

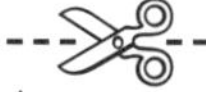

These questions guide you through the topic. If you need help to answer them, look at pages 172–177 of the Collins textbook.

10.4 short **questions** and **activities**

1. What ethical principles are enshrined in the Department of Health's Research Governance Framework for Health and Social Care (2005, Second Edition)?
2. Identify at least three groups of people who have been the victims of unethical medical research.
3. What was the real aim of the Milgram Obedience Study?
4. What was the real aim of the Stanford Prison Study?
5. Identify three examples of health research that are likely to involve a degree of risk to the research participants.
6. Name two examples of care research that have led to more distributive justice.

10.4 summary worksheet

RESEARCH ETHICS

With regard to the issue of ethics in research, identify three similarities and three differences between the Milgram Obedience Study and the Stanford Prison Study.

Similarities

- ...
- ...
- ...

Differences

- ...
- ...
- ...

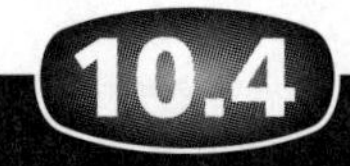

extension**activity**sheet

SCIENCE AND CONSCIENCE

'Science without conscience is the ruin of the soul.'

(Rabelais, 1532)

a Write down what you understand this statement to mean.

b Explain how this statement could relate to care research and care practice and/or policy.

c To what extent do you believe that this statement is a true one?

10.5 Quantitative research

The rationale behind this topic is to show how vital it is in care research to count and measure data. How, for example, can we implement shorter hospital waiting lists if we do not know current average waiting times? Or how can we decide who is poor if we do not establish an official poverty line?

Quantitative research rightly sets high standards for precision, and this helps care practitioners and care policy-makers to develop carefully planned interventions. A quantitative design also makes it easier to calculate the effects of particular measures, such as the impact of a healthy living campaign on young smokers.

Answers to the *Check your understanding* questions on page 183 of the Collins textbook.

1 Quantitative data are data in the form of numbers. These data address quantitative issues, such as the average time it takes from GP referral to consultation with a hip replacement surgeon in Wales, or investigating the statistical link between high alcohol intake and liver disease.

2 Quantitative data in the form of inferential statistics can help care researchers to assess the effects of care interventions. Inferential statistics can be used, for example, to assess the effects of an intervention to improve the mobility of wheelchair users in a city centre.

3 Close-ended questions in survey research enable researchers to quantify and analyse (using statistics) the responses of survey respondents, e.g. how many women, compared to men, are on low incomes?

4 Similarities: both methods are quantitative; both investigate effects through the use of a pre-test and a post-test. Differences: the true experiment requires random assignment of respondents to experimental and control groups, whereas the quasi-experiment does not; the true experiment obtains a greater level of control over variables, compared to the quasi-experiment.

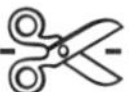

These questions guide you through the topic. If you need help to answer them, look at pages 178–183 of the Collins textbook.

10.5 short **questions** and **activities**

1 How do statisticians define a 'population'?

2 What is the connection between a representative random sample and a slice of pie?

3 How do quantitative questionnaires and quantitative interviews resemble and differ from each other?

4 What type of question is a 'circle one' question in a questionnaire?

5 What is the essential feature of all experiments in quantitative research?

6 What are the three main types of clinical trial?

10.5 summary worksheet

METHODS AND RESEARCH TOPICS

Methods
• Close-ended interview
• True experiment
• Quasi-experiment

Research topics
• Comparing the effects of two different medications
• Comparing the effects of two different anti-poverty measures
• Conducting a patient-satisfaction survey

Above is a list of research methods, and a list of research topics.

a Explain, in your own words, what each research method involves.

Close-ended interview ....

....

....

True experiment ....

....

....

Quasi-experiment ....

....

....

b Match the best research method to each research topic, and briefly justify your choice.

CONSTRUCTING A QUESTIONNAIRE

In quantitative research, questionnaires and interviews often use a closed-question design – using questions of the 'circle one' (single-coded) kind, such as:

How many pints of beer did you drink yesterday? (*circle one*)

none 1 2 3 4 5 6 or more

Using the above question as an example, construct a closed-question questionnaire (up to 10 questions) on a topic related to health and social care, and try it out on some of the students in your class. Then report your findings in the form of concise descriptive statistics.

10.6 Qualitative research

The rationale behind this topic is to impress upon students the need to produce data that are rich in first-hand testimony. The aim here is to get at the 'text' behind the numbers – for example, the voice of social work clients as well as how many of them receive homecare.

Some students (and some researchers for that matter!) seem to think that research methods should be *either* qualitative *or* quantitative. This is not a tenable position because the investigation of complex data requires a range of methods. Students therefore need to learn to work with both text and number.

Answers to the *Check your understanding* questions on page 187 of the Collins textbook.

1 **Qualitative data are data that are typically in the form of words. These data reveal the 'text' of an issue, such as how cancer patients express their hopes and fears in their own words.**

2 **Qualitative data, expressed as patients' own words about their treatment, can help care researchers to understand nuances that are not easily captured in numbers. For example, when a patient says, 'I want to be more involved in decisions about what treatment works best for me and my family', this conveys a concern about patient autonomy that might easily be lost in a bare statistic.**

3 **A good qualitative interview guide strikes the right balance between identifying relevant themes while at the same time leaving space for significant leads that might arise during the course of the interview. Leads that the interviewee initiates can be particularly useful because they may raise important issues that the interviewer may not have thought about before.**

4 **A mix of quantitative and qualitative methods can produce detailed, rich data by combining number and text, such as the extent of homelessness in a particular community and the personal pain of being on the streets.**

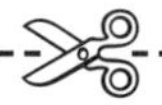

These questions guide you through the topic. If you need help to answer them, look at pages 184–187 of the Collins textbook.

10.6 short **questions** and **activities**

1. What does it mean to 'clarify' an interview transcript?
2. What is an open-ended interview?
3. What is the function of an interview guide?
4. What is full immersion observation?
5. Referring to a concrete care issue, show how the use of qualitative data can provide a ressearcher with important information.
6. What is meant by the term 'mixed toolbag'?

summary worksheet

METHODS AND RESEARCH TOPICS

Methods
• Open-ended interview • Full immersion observation • Complete separation observation

Research topics
• Watching other colleagues on a ward round • Watching audio-visual recordings of interactions between social workers and their clients • Eliciting patients' perceptions of how they are treated by health care professionals

Above is a list of research methods and a list of research topics.

a Explain, in your own words, what each research method involves.

Open-ended interview ....

....

....

Full immersion observation

....

....

....

Complete separation observation

....

....

....

b Match the best research method to each research topic, and briefly justify your choice.

extension**activity**sheet

CONSTRUCTING AN INTERVIEW GUIDE

One way of maintaining a balance between staying on track and going where the respondent leads is to use an 'interview guide'. This is a basic checklist of themes within which the interviewer is able to explore and probe particular issues while still being able to pursue relevant leads as and when they arise. An interview guide helps to ensure that the same general areas of inquiry are pursued with each person interviewed.

Construct an interview guide that could be used to find out what young people think about doing regular exercise. Try the guide out on three students in your class, and present your findings in the form of major themes (or categories, as they are also called).

10.7 Census and epidemiological data

The rationale behind this topic is to help students to appreciate the importance of patterns in what are mainly quantitative data. The patterns (typically relationships between variables, such as between poverty and health) are not always apparent, so they have to be looked for.

Given that Census and epidemiological data often apply to local and national care issues, these data are especially relevant when making evidence-based policy decisions.

Answers to the *Check your understanding* questions on page 191 of the Collins textbook.

1 Similarities: data from both sources assist care practitioners and policy-makers in planning, implementing and evaluating; both sources provide statistics on the state of the nation.
Differences: Census data address a broad range of issues, whereas epidemiological data focus on the specific area of patterns of disease in human, animal and plant populations; being a survey of all households in the nation, the Census provides data from a total headcount, whereas epidemiological research typically produces data that are based on representative samples.

2 Dr John Snow deservedly enjoys the status of a pioneer in epidemiology because his research, *On the Mode of Communication of Cholera* (1849), has inspired other researchers to gather and use epidemiological information to prevent and manage diseases.

3 Census and epidemiological data show that healthy eating leads to good physical health and that unhealthy eating has the opposite effect. If heeded, this evidence might encourage policy-makers to fund healthy school dinners, thereby helping children to benefit from at least one healthy meal a day.

4 Census and epidemiological studies not only investigate large statistical populations, they also examine statistical links between multiple variables. For these reasons, methods that produce quantitative data are the logical choice – at least, in most cases.

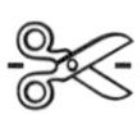

These questions guide you through the topic. If you need help to answer them, look at pages 188–191 of the Collins textbook.

10.7 short questions and activities

1. What is the Census?
2. Identify three examples of Census data that might interest care researchers, and explain why.
3. Identify a current epidemiological crisis, and briefly describe it.
4. What was the reasoning behind Dr John Snow's epidemiological investigation in London?
5. Is Dr John Snow justifiably regarded as a pioneer in the field of epidemiology?

summaryworksheet

HEALTH TRENDS

The main results of the 2001 Census are available free on the Office for National Statistics (ONS) website.

a Go online and locate the site. Write down the web address.

b Then find an example of a health trend that has been identified over a period of years.

i What is the trend you have chosen to investigate further?

ii Write a brief summary of this trend, and present your findings in a short report.

KICKING THE HABIT

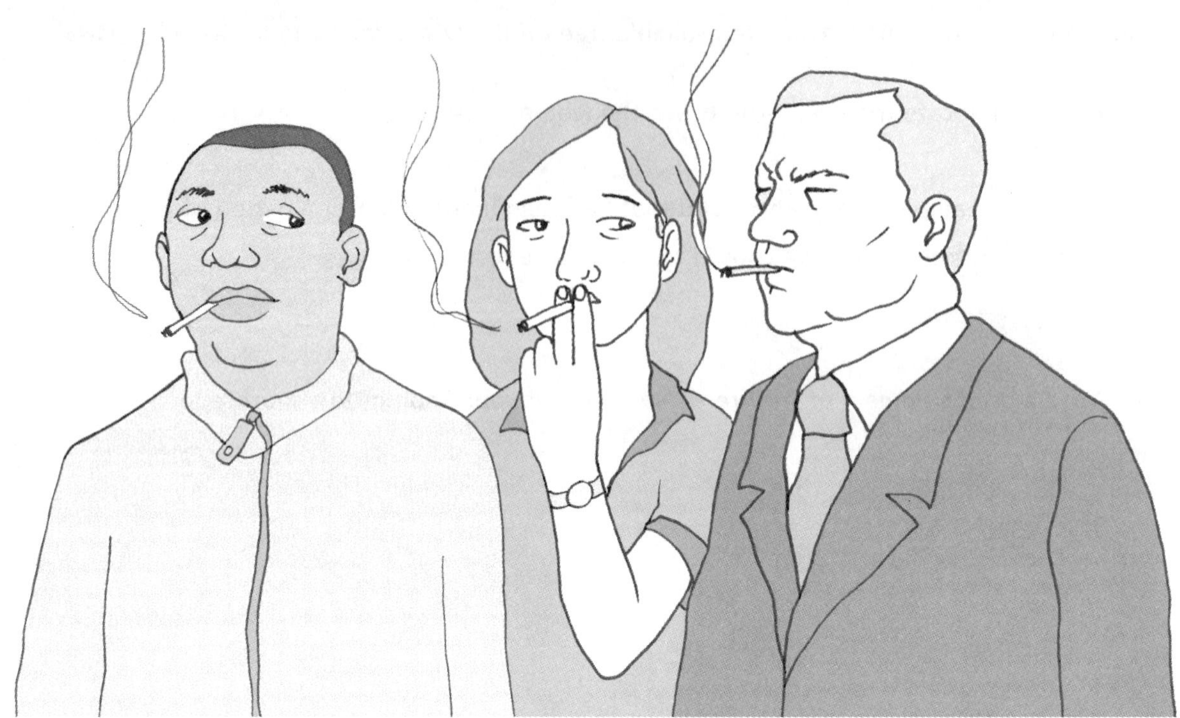

Imagine that you are going to address a group of adult smokers who want to stop smoking. Assume that most of them are laypersons. Your task is to help them kick the habit and not to resume it later.

Using appropriate Census and epidemiological data, prepare a talk that is creative, scientific, easy-to-understand and, above all, persuasive. You may wish to do this as a Powerpoint presentation.

Try out your talk on an audience of students and teachers.

10.8 Care research and public policy

The rationale behind this topic is to argue the case for a care research agenda that flows into public policy. Max Weber's rebuke of an indifferent social science is a relevant thought.

Even though the government says that it wants to use research findings to improve public policy, it is relevant to highlight some of the tensions that arise when heated political emotion confronts sober scientific rationality. Students might also want to consider how their own political views might influence the way that they conduct research and how they interpret published research findings.

Answers to the *Check your understanding* questions on page 195 of the Collins textbook.

1 'Inclusive design' refers to the designing of products and environments so that *everyone* can use them, without the need for adaptation. 'Independent living' is a human rights philosophy which maintains that people who are disabled have the right to live with dignity and with appropriate support in their own homes, to participate fully in their communities and to have control over their lives.

2 The Strategy Unit of the government provides policy-makers with strategic evidence-based advice on major policy issues. Based on this research, the government knows, for example, that disabled people are more likely to face diminished life chances, compared to people who are not disabled. This finding has triggered a series of policy interventions, one of which is action to develop the inclusive design of products, services and environments so that people of all 'abilities' and ages are able to use them in their everyday lives.

Another 'think tank', the National Centre for Social Research, conducts research that has been guiding health and social policy debates for several decades. Findings from its largest survey, the annual *Health Survey for England* (which tracks the health of the nation), are used to improve the targeting of national health policies.

3 Emotions can compromise policy decisions if feelings ride roughshod over rational thinking. This is not to suggest that conviction politics, fired by heated emotions, are necessarily irrational. But they can be, especially if a war of words flies in the face of the best argument.

4 Inclusive design helps people who are disabled to gain more self-determination in society, thereby promoting – and being inextricably linked to – independent living.

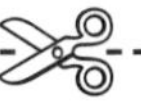

These questions guide you through the topic. If you need help to answer them, look at pages 192–195 of the Collins textbook.

10.8 short **questions** and **activities**

1. Why should politicians consult care research data?
2. Identify two 'think tanks' and briefly describe their role in public policy.
3. 'Evidence shows that reductions in the incidence and severity of disability in a population can be achieved by improving performance via modifying features of the social and physical environment.' Put this sentence into plain English and illustrate it with a concrete example.
4. Provide three examples of inclusive design (existing or proposed) that are not mentioned in this unit.
5. What does it mean, to say that 'poor life chance outcomes are both a cause and a result of disability'?
6. What is the essential promise of evidence-based policy in health and social care?

summaryworksheet

PLANNED WELL-BEING

On page 193, the authors identify three examples (Rowntree, Webb and Townsend) of scientific research in the service of health and social care. The examples date from the early 20th century to the early 21st century.

a Identify three more examples for each of the three centuries in the table below.

	Example of research serving health and social care
19th century	
20th century	
21st century	

b Choose *one* of the examples you identified and write down what the findings of the research were.

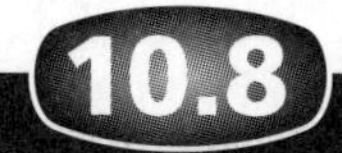

extension**activity**sheet

PUTTING RESEARCH TO USE

Unfortunately, there is no guarantee that good research will be put to effective use. Indeed one of the most important studies of health inequalities in the UK, the *Black Report* of 1980, just sat on library bookshelves instead of provoking the action that was needed to put things right.

Investigate the reasons behind the relative failure of policy-makers to act upon the findings of the *Black Report*. Present your conclusions in a short report.

10.9 Doing your own research

The main aim of this topic is to help students to carry out a small investigation well, and always with their own safety and well-being and those of the people whom they study firmly at the forefront. If students do not personally know potential research participants, then it is essential that the students only contact persons whom the teacher approves. This is an important safeguard for the students.

This topic gives advice and guidance for students on how to conduct a small-scale research project. Their project is, in itself, enough to get on with so, apart from the *Check your understanding* answers, we have not included here the other activities that feature in Topics 1–8.

Answers to the *Check your understanding* questions on page 199 of the Collins textbook.

1 **All researchers (including *you*) have an ethical duty to respect and protect the rights and safety of those whom they study. Furthermore, all researchers (including *you*) have an obligation and the right to protect their own personal safety when they carry out an investigation.**

2 **Research involving a hypothesis seeks to find out if a preconceived idea stands up to hard evidence, whereas exploratory research aims to find out what hard evidence reveals without having any prior ideas.**

3 **I could carry out an attitude survey of students in my year at my school or college. For example, I could seek to find out how many (and what percentage of) students in a representative sample think (ranging from totally agree to totally disagree) about ten proposed statements concerning healthy living. I would use a self-administered questionnaire with closed questions and a rating scale. In my introduction, I would present a short systematic review (based on an internet search) of young people's views on healthy living.**

In defence of my choices:

- **Using a sample of students from my school or college is safer than approaching strangers.**
- **It is relatively straightforward to randomly select a sample of students in my year.**
- **A closed-question questionnaire could yield relevant, quantifiable data.**
- **A systematic review of relevant studies would place my specific research questions and findings into a wider context, and might permit a degree of comparison.**

4 **The Discussion part of a research report should contain my interpretation of the data (that is, what the data suggest) and any potential uses to which my findings could be put (e.g., identifying possible steps to improve healthy living through whole school/college policies). I should also state any limitations that might affect the reliability and validity of my findings.**

The reasons for my thinking are:

- **A discussion allows room for making sense of the data.**
- **A discussion customarily invites the researcher to consider good practice implications.**
- **No research is perfect, so honesty about limitations helps readers to make a more informed judgement about the researcher's findings and conclusions.**

Doing your own research: preliminary preparation

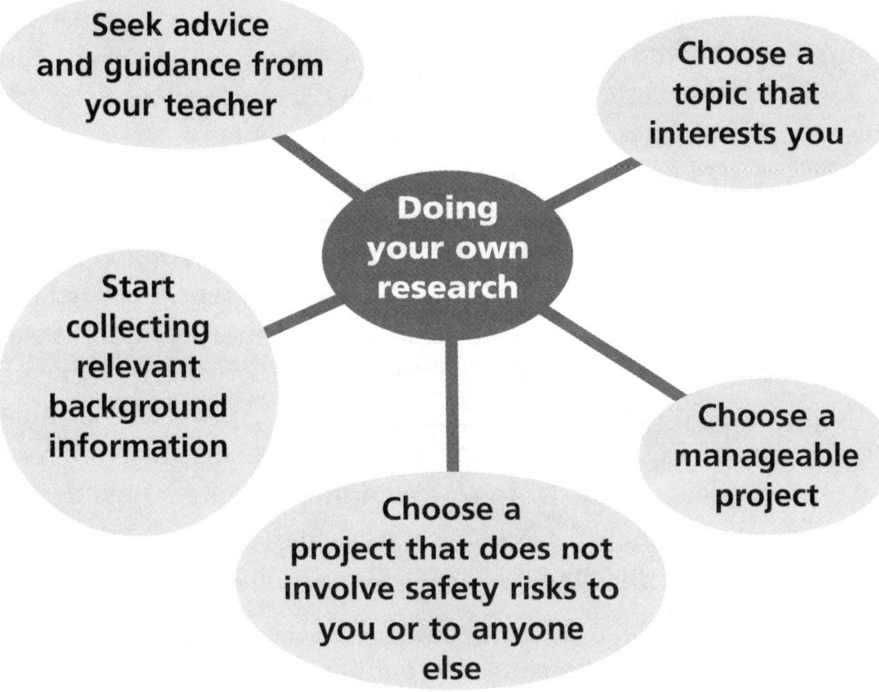

Main steps in a systematic review

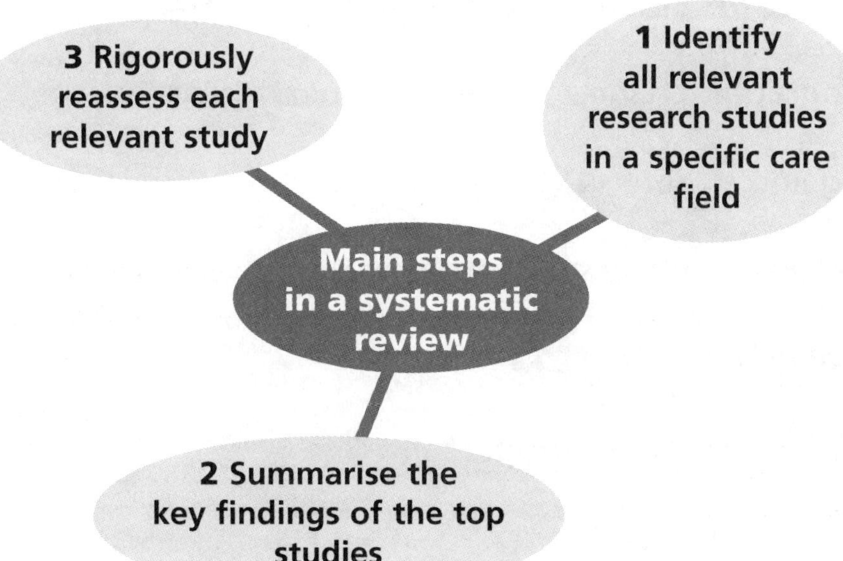

Social Issues and Welfare Needs is a portfolio-tested unit and will require students to produce a written report on a social issue or welfare need of interest to them. The social issue or welfare need should affect at least one of the following client groups: people who are ill, young children, older people, and people with specific needs. In the report, the students should cover the origins of the social issue of welfare need they are investigating, and any related demographic changes, together with its contemporary nature, and government responses in terms of policy. To achieve high marks, the report will need to be accurate, clear, detailed and well-explained. The students should show very good skills in obtaining information, drawn from a wide range of different types of sources. The students should show excellent understanding of demographic factors and explanations of data. They should show very good analytical skills, make relevant and extensive links to work-related issues and show an excellent level of evaluative skills. They should demonstrate a high degree of independence in their work. Whatever level a student is working at, they should follow the specific help given in the assessment guidance section of the specification.

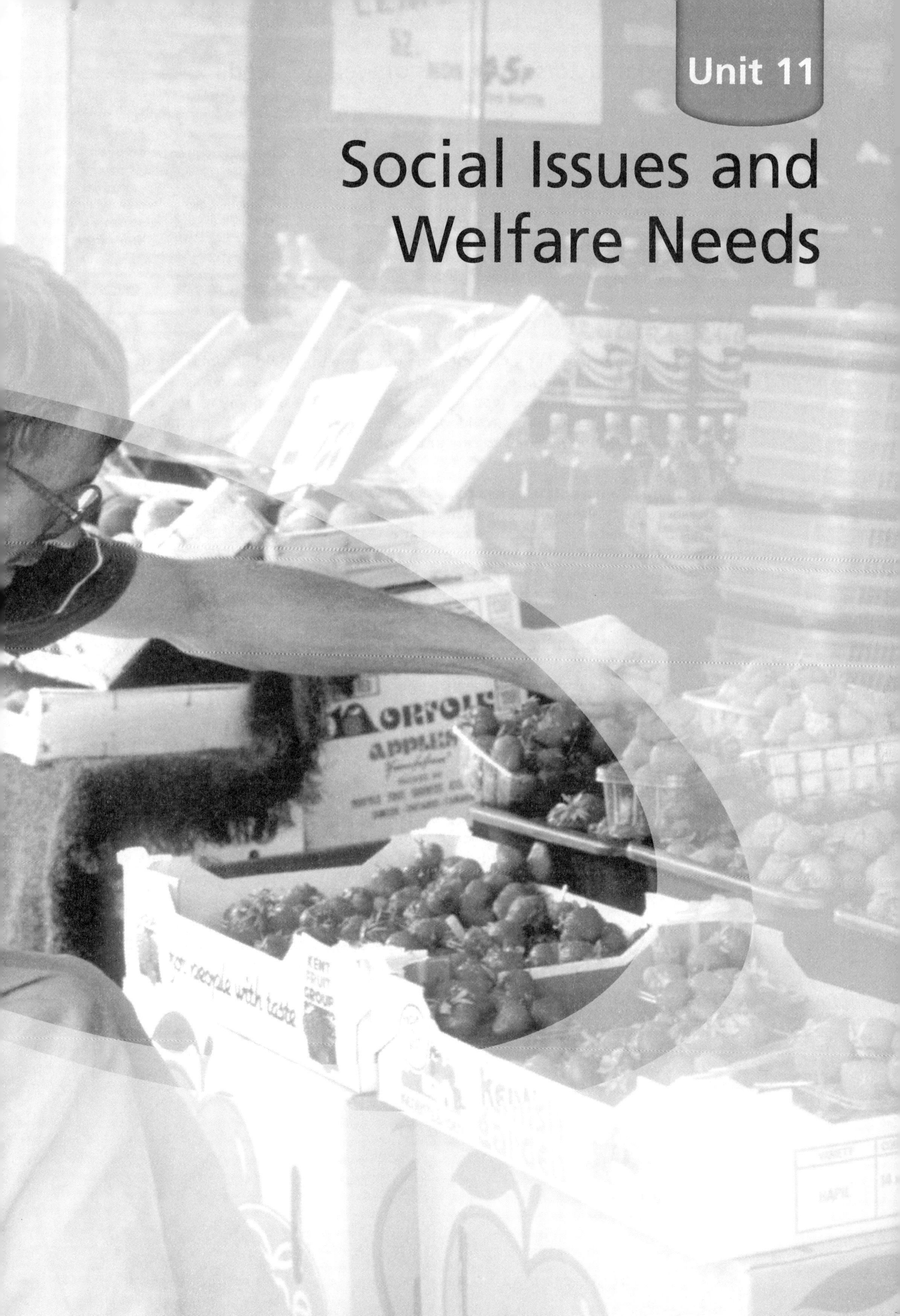

Unit 11

Social Issues and Welfare Needs

11.1 Social factors and areas of welfare need

This topic provides an introduction to different approaches to the care and support of the vulnerable in society. In all societies there are groups of people who are potentially vulnerable, including children, young people and the frail elderly. Whether they are supported and how they are supported, however, varies from society to society and at different times in history. In some societies it is the responsibility of the individual and their family. In others, the community plays a key role, and in many societies of the twenty-first century the state is central in the provision of care and welfare.

Getting you thinking helps students to focus on these general issues of welfare. Through discussion of the questions, students will consider where responsibility for the vulnerable should lie. Should this be with the individual and their family or should the state provide protection 'from the cradle to the grave'?

Answers to the *Check your understanding* questions on page 205 of the Collins textbook.

1 **'Laissez- faire' describes a view that the government should not interfere in the workings of the economy nor in the provision of welfare services. The government should 'leave well alone'. In a laissez-faire economy there would be few if any state-provided welfare services. Individuals and their families would be required to care and support each other, in good times and in bad.**

2 **The term 'welfare state' refers to a society where the government takes responsibility and makes provision for the health and welfare of the nation. It was a term first used during the 1940s following the publication of the Beveridge Report and it normally refers to the key services established at this time, including the National Health Service, the social security systems and state-funded education, housing and other social services.**

3 **The five giants identified in the Beveridge Report were: Want, Disease, Squalor, Idleness, and Ignorance. Students may have used more up to date language, such as poverty, ill-health, poor housing, unemployment and lack of education, but they should also be familiar with Beveridge's own terms. This was a very important report in British social and economic history and it is appropriate to use and explain the terms of the day.**

4 **It is argued that a dependency culture may develop as a result of a welfare state because people may rely on state services and other benefits rather than working hard and taking full responsibility for their own lives. They may not 'save for a rainy day', or provide care for older relatives, for example, because they regard this as the government's responsibility. There is often a judgement associated with this view that people will depend on the state too much. They may claim benefits rather than work.**

5 **'The New Right' is a term associated with the views of Mrs Thatcher, Prime Minister during the 1980s. This view holds that the government should play a minimal role in the provision of welfare. Taxes should be low and people should decide how they spend their money, making their own provision for health and welfare needs. Students may have identified the similarity between the New Right views and the laissez-faire of the nineteenth century.**

These questions guide you through the topic. If you need help to answer them, look at pages 202–205 of the Collins textbook.

11.1 short questions and activities

1. Describe two different approaches that societies may take in meeting the needs of the vulnerable.
2. Describe two types of poor relief available through the Poor Law provision.
3. Briefly describe the social and economic changes that were taking place at the time of the 'liberal reforms' and identify three welfare reforms introduced by the Liberal government (1905–1915).
4. List Beveridge's 'five giant evils' and provide a twenty-first-century synonym for each.
5. Describe welfare measures introduced shortly after the Second World War to address each of the 'five evil giants'.
6. Briefly describe the approach to welfare of
   - The New Right
   - The Third Way approach to welfare provision.

summary worksheet

CHANGES IN THE PROVISION OF CARE

Mrs Brothers is 85 and lives quite independently in a small and comfortable flat in the north of England. She has three adult children, one is in Australia and the other two, who are both married, live in London. Her GP's surgery is nearby. She has meals-on-wheels delivered three days a week, and a home care assistant visits her once a week to help with household chores. This is very different from her childhood memories. Her grandparents lived in the countryside. There were no pensions, they had to pay to see the doctor, they had to find the rent for their house and there was certainly no meals-on-wheels. While her grandfather was working they had managed to pay their bills. They had saved a bit of money too, but this money ran out – and in the end they were forced to go and live in the workhouse to survive.

a Why, according to the text, did Mrs Brothers' grandparent end up in a workhouse?

b Identify five reasons why it was seen as necessary for governments to provide some health and care services in the early years of the twentieth century.

1

2

3

4

5

c Why could the approach to Mrs Brother's care be seen as an example of community care ?

d Identify two arguments in favour and two against community care provision for older people.

Arguments in favour

1

2

Arguments against

1

2

extension**activity**sheet

RESPONSES TO HOMELESSNESS

Until recently, Tom, who is nineteen, lived with his mother. But when she married Frank last year, Tom and his new stepfather did not get on. There were numerous arguments at home and eventually this led to Tom walking out. He has been sleeping on a friend's sofa for a few weeks, but now he has to move on. He has nowhere to go – but he won't go back home.

a Describe the possible response to such problems by governments adopting the following approaches to welfare:

i An interventionist, welfare state approach

ii The New Right.

b Discuss the strengths and limitations of each approach for Tom and his family.

11.2 Demographic change and welfare need

This topic introduces students to the main sources of demographic data and the central concerns of demographers. The extent of changes in the size and structure of the population and the reasons for those changes are discussed. Students will consider the reasons for the changes in the birth rate and the death rate in the UK, particularly during the last century, and also issues of immigration and emigration.

The *Getting you thinking* questions should stimulate discussion on changes in the size and structure of the family, the institution with which, arguably, the students are most familiar. Students should consider how far the image in the textbook and that portrayed in the media is of the typical family in modern Britain. This will inform discussion later in this unit on how changes in the family may lead to changes in the provision of health and care services.

Answers to the *Check your understanding* questions on page 211 of the Collins textbook.

1 **The most likely reasons for the fall in the birth rate during the twentieth century are**

(i) improved methods of contraception
(ii) the greater availability of contraceptives
(iii) women choosing work and a career over large families
(iv) the high cost of child rearing
(v) the increased value placed on a high standard of living.

You may have considered that the development of a welfare state may mean that people do not need to have large families in order to be cared for in old age. It is expected that there will be state-supported services to meet these needs.

2 **The most likely reasons for the fall in the death rate during the twentieth century are:**

- **The improved public health systems, e.g. clean water, improved sewerage, immunisation schemes.**
- **Much improved medical knowledge.**
- **The introduction of a national health service.**
- **Improved health and safety practices in industry.**
- **Improved standards of living, leading to better and warmer housing, better diets.**
- **Better maternity and post-natal care, leading to a fall in both infant mortality and the death of mothers during pregnancy and childbirth.**

3 **Infant mortality rates may reflect the levels of social and economic progress because the factors linked with high infant mortality (e.g. unclean water and poor sewerage, poor maternity care, inadequate child immunisation programmes, insufficient access to health services, poor housing and poor diets) are themselves associated with poverty and a depressed economy. Good public health provision and effective health care is essential for a growing modern economy.**

4 **Net migration refers to the difference between the numbers emigrating (leaving a country to live elsewhere) and those immigrating (entering the country with a view to living there).**

5 **Reasons why people may choose to emigrate include:**

- **The need to find work**
- **Escaping poverty**
- **The chance to improve their standard of living**
- **Escaping political or religious persecution – many refugees are fleeing to avoid such persecution**
- **Personal reasons for 'making a new start'.**

These questions guide you through the topic. If you need help to answer them, look at pages 206–211 of the Collins textbook.

11.2 short **questions** and **activities**

1. Define the term 'demography'.
2. Changes in the size of the population are caused by natural changes in the population and by emigration and immigration. Define these terms.
3. Why may governments use Census data and other demographic information?
4. Why is it important to always identify the source of demographic information?
5. What is meant by the term 'dependent population'?

summary worksheet

POPULATION TRENDS

Mrs Lee is 87 and has a new great-grandson – Joshua, born last May. Mrs Lee has two adult children, four grandchildren – and now a great-grandson. This is very different from the family structure she knew as a child. Mrs Lee had been one of ten children. Two of her siblings died as babies. She never knew her grandparents. Both of her grandfathers were miners who had died before she was born. Both of her grandmothers died before she started school at the age of five. Her own parents had died in their seventies. Now there were four generations in the family, and her friends were sharing similar stories.

a Give three reasons for the differences in size of the family over the generations described.

1 ....

2 ....

3 ....

b Give three reasons for the different age structure of the families described in the case study.

1 ....

2 ....

3 ....

c Referring to the 'Immigration and emigration' graph on page 210:

i Identify two trends in immigration and emigration in the period 1995–2004.

....

ii Calculate the level of net migration in 2004.

....

d Identify and explain four possible reasons for these trends.

1 ....

2 ....

3 ....

4 ....

extension**activity**sheet

DEMOGRAPHIC CHANGE

a Referring to the 'Changes in the death rate' graph on page 208, describe the differences in the death rates of men and women between 1901 and 2003.

b Discuss the impact of demographic changes on the care needs of a society.

c Compare the impact of a New Right approach to care needs as opposed to the 'Third Way' proposed by recent Labour governments.

11.3 An ageing society

This topic, building on the previous topic on demographic change, considers further the implications – for the care and support of older people – of an ageing population and changes in family structure. Students are introduced to up-to-date statistical evidence and current social policy and practice in this area to inform their study.

The image and questions posed at the beginning of the topic aim to consider and challenge stereotypical ideas and views of older people and, building on that discussion, for students to consider the range of health and welfare services that may meet their needs.

Answers to the *Check your understanding* questions on page 215 of the Collins textbook.

1 **The term 'community care' refers to provision where people are cared for in their homes or in small 'family' units rather than in large, less personal institutions. Students may well give examples to support their answers, e.g. sheltered housing complexes for older people, home care services, or residential support for people with learning difficulties or mental health problems in small domestic units for five or six residents. The contrast is with large, hospital-type care.**

2 **Community care services that may be provided for older people who need support with daily living activities include: home care assistants, home helps or other domiciliary care support, meals on wheels, district nurse services, occupational therapy, physiotherapy, plus the GP and other services of the local health centre. Students may also have mentioned the support of informal carers, especially family, friends and neighbours.**

3 **There may be poverty in older age because of a large drop in income on retiring from work. People who began work shortly after the Second World War may not have made provision for retirement beyond their national insurance contributions to their state pension. They understood that they and their families would be cared for by a welfare state. They would be cared for 'from the cradle to the grave'. People who have had interrupted employment – because of redundancy, for example, or for health or family reasons – or have earned poor wages or had no occupational pension are most likely to suffer poverty in old age. The state pension is increasingly inadequate to keep people out of relative poverty.**

4 **In the twenty-first century it may be difficult for adult children to provide practical care for older relatives because families are smaller and because children are less likely to live close to older relatives than was the case in previous generations. Women, who traditionally have been the carers, are more likely to work than was the case in the past. There is little financial help to support children who are looking after older relatives, and employers are not required to be sympathetic – there is no statutory 'carers leave'. Further housing policy has not addressed the needs of extended families in caring for older relatives and friends.**

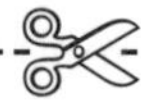

These questions guide you through the topic. If you need help to answer them, look at pages 212–215 of the Collins textbook.

11.3 short **questions** and **activities**

1 Using the information provided in this topic, outline the evidence for the claim that we live in an ageing society.

2 Using the information provided in this topic, what evidence is there to suggest that attitudes to older people vary from society to society?

3 Identify one way in which the European Union is promoting equality for older people.

4 Outline the changes in our society which may have led to a need for a wide range of care services for older people.

5 How have care services for older people changed in the past hundred years?

11.3 summary worksheet

SUPPORT FOR AN AGEING POPULATION

Referring to the 'Under 16s and people aged 65 and over' graph on page 208:

a Approximately how many people in the UK population were over 65 in 1971?

b Approximately what is the population of people over 65 predicted for 2021?

c Compare the difference in the number of people under 16 and the number over 65 in 1971 with the difference predicted for 2021

d What is the demographic term used to describe the populations of the UK who are under 16 and over 65? (You may need to refer to the 'key terms' section in Topic 2.)

e Explain the possible consequences of these population trends for care of older people in our society. Compare your ideas with those identified by other members of your group.

LIFESTYLES IN OLDER AGE

Sally, who is 14, has four grandparents all of whom are retired and in their late sixties. Sally's mum's parents seem to be having the time of their life. They were both doctors and had a good income all their life and now have a good occupational pension. They have a beautiful home. They play golf, go on holiday abroad during the winter, take their grandchildren away during the summer holidays – and really, they just don't seem to age.

Sally's dad's parents, however, are not doing quite so well. Granddad was a steelworker and was made redundant in the 1970s. He managed to get other jobs but they were all poorly paid and there was no occupational pension. Grandma worked part-time as a cleaner but she didn't have a works pension either and she never paid in to the state pension scheme. They still live in the council house that they moved to when they got married. It is damp and difficult to heat. Sally knows that in the winter her Dad's parents have to choose between spending their small pensions on eating well or keeping warm. They do manage to go away on holiday for a week in the summer, but they have never been on holiday abroad.

a Describe the differences between Sally's two sets of grandparents in terms of lifestyle and quality of life.

b Discuss the possible impact of these differences on their health, well-being and life expectancy. Refer to relevant research to inform and support your discussion.

Discrimination and access to health and care services

This focus of this topic is equality and diversity and their impact on the provision of and access to health and care services. There is discussion of the impact of current legislation and associated European Union directives on policy and practice in the UK.

Through consideration of the scenario described in the *Getting you thinking* section, the setting up of a new nursery, students will be required to consider their own attitudes to equality and diversity, especially multi-cultural issues and the role of men as childcare professionals. They may use this as a preparation for discussion of current policy and practice in this area.

Answers to the *Check your understanding* questions on page 221 of the Collins textbook.

1 'Prejudice' is holding preconceived opinions and attitudes towards particular groups which are not modified in the light of new experiences that might contradict your view. 'Discrimination' is when a person is treated differently, and in this context normally less favourably, on the grounds of particular characteristics, e.g. race, gender, sexual orientation or age. Discriminatory behaviour often arises from prejudicial attitudes. A 'stereotype' is an over-simplified image or idea about the characteristics of a particular group, e.g. 'women are better at childcare than men' or 'all negroes are good at sport and they have a good sense of rhythm'. Stereotypes can often lead to prejudicial attitudes. 'Diversity' in this context refers to the wide range of different cultural groups in our society and the different customs, religious practices and forms of celebration that they bring.

2 It is necessary to understand individual differences when supporting people in health and care settings in order to: understand and meet their individual care needs; ensure that they are not misunderstood; and to ensure that they fully understand the provision and services available. Students may have given examples, e.g. it is important to understand the dress and dietary customs of different cultural and religious groups, or to appreciate the customary roles for men and women in different social groups, because misunderstanding or lack of knowledge could lead to embarrassment or offence and might limit access to the service. It is necessary to understand individual differences in order that everyone can be treated with equal respect and care.

3 The Sex Discrimination Act 1975 protects people from discrimination on the grounds of sex and marital status. The Race Relations Act 1976 protects people from discrimination on the grounds of race, colour, nationality and national or ethnic origin. The Disability Discrimination Act 1995 protects people with disabilities and learning difficulties, and the Special Educational Needs and Disabilities Act (SENDA) 2001 protects people in education and training. Students may have also mentioned that the European Union Equal Treatment Directive 2000 protects people throughout the EU from discrimination on the grounds of religion, age and sexual orientation.

4 Direct discrimination within English law refers to treating a person less favourably on grounds of their sex or race, e.g. requiring that a bar attendant should be female, or a caretaker male, or a secretary white.

Indirect discrimination consists of imposing conditions – which are not relevant to a job – that would be a barrier for some groups of people, e.g. advertising a plumbing course for all but providing no toilet facilities for women and no learning provision for women needing maternity leave.

5 **There are currently three equality commissions in Great Britain – the Commission for Racial Equality, the Equal Opportunities Commission and the Disability Rights Commission – and in Northern Ireland there is the Equality Commission Northern Ireland. They have a general remit to promote equality of opportunity for the group they represent. The commissions will provide advice and information to individuals, employers and service providers, support people in getting their rights under the laws, publish research and conduct high-profile campaigns to promote equal rights, and investigate companies and organisations where unlawful practice is persistent and take legal action where this is necessary.**

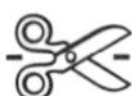

These questions guide you through the topic. If you need help to answer them, look at pages 216–221 of the Collins textbook.

11.4 short **questions** and **activities**

1. Explain the difference between prejudice and discrimination.
2. Why may stereotyping an individual or group lead to discrimination?
3. Explain the difference between the ideas of 'equality of access' to services and 'equality of outcomes'.
4. Identify two differences, other than their client group, between the requirements of the Race Relations Act 1976 and the Disability Discrimination Act 1995 .
5. Identify the consequences for equality law in the United Kingdom of the European Union Equal Treatment Directives.
6. What is the new role for the proposed Commission for Equality and Human Rights?

summaryworksheet

DISABILITY AND EMPLOYMENT

Lola worked as a clerical assistant in a medium-sized engineering company. Following a serious car accident on holiday she needed to use a wheelchair at work. The company were initially sympathetic but then gave her notice that she was being made redundant. The premises, they said, were not suited to wheelchair users. Lola knew about the Disability Discrimination Act (1995) and contacted her local Citizens' Advice Bureau (CAB). The CAB wrote to the company on her behalf pointing out their responsibilities to 'make reasonable adjustments to their premises' for people with disabilities. They reminded the company that Lola had the right to take her case to an employment tribunal should she consider their response to be discriminatory.

a Identify six other areas of discrimination covered by the law in the UK.

1 ....

2 ....

3 ....

4 ....

5 ....

6 ....

b Identify three other areas of discrimination that are not covered by legislation.

1 ....

2 ....

3 ....

Compare your list with other members of your class. Do you think that the law should cover these additional areas?

c Describe three reasonable adjustments that a company could make to their premises where there was currently no wheelchair access.

1 ....

....

2 ....

....

3 ....

....

d How might the Disability Rights Commission support Lola in securing her rights?

....

....

....

e Identify two strengths and two weaknesses of the Disability Discrimination Act in securing individual rights.

Strengths ....

....

Weaknesses ....

....

extension**activity**sheet

THE EQUALITY LEGISLATION

a Discuss how far equality legislation has been successful in securing the rights of people from disadvantaged groups.

b Positive discrimination could be described as 'a policy of providing disadvantaged groups with additional rights, resources or opportunities to combat a history of discrimination'. Discuss the advantages and disadvantages of such a policy.

11.5 An unequal society

This topic is closely linked with the previous discussion of discrimination. It focuses on issues of inequality, and particularly economic inequalities. Students are introduced to the concepts of social stratification, social class and social exclusion, together with their impact on individual life chances and their associated health and well-being.

The *Getting you thinking* section provides a context for an initial discussion of students' perceptions of our society. 'Are we all middle class now? Are there opportunities for us all to succeed if we are willing to work hard?' They may find it helpful to make brief notes of this discussion and revisit them when they have completed the topic. Are the views sustainable in the light of the evidence?

Answers to the *Check your understanding* questions on page 225 of the Collins textbook.

1 **'Social stratification' refers to the ranking of people according to their status within the society. 'Social class' is one form of social stratification. There are, however, many definitions of social class. Common to most is the view that position in society is determined by our economic circumstances, which will then influence our life choices, our opportunities and future prospects. 'Social exclusion' is a term used to describe a situation where people are unable to participate fully in society for a number of related reasons, often including poverty, unemployment, poor housing or homelessness, poor health and poor educational achievement.**

2 **The Social Exclusion Unit was set up to provide a coordinated solution to a range of social problems, including high levels of crime, poor school attendance, high unemployment and perceived unemployability, homelessness and little participation in the social and political life of the community.**

3 **Prejudice may lead to discriminatory behaviour because prejudicial attitudes are not easily changed by rational arguments. When these strongly held views and feelings are directed towards disadvantaged groups it is a small step for them to manifest themselves in conscious or unconscious discriminatory behaviour. If we have negative attitudes towards a particular group we are likely to be wary of them and treat them less favourably than other members of society.**

4 **A stereotype is a set of characteristics that members of a particular group are said to possess, e.g. that people from particular estates are in debt and lazy and their children are in the lowest groups at school. When a stereotype is widely held, it is sometimes said that the group have been 'labelled'. These characteristics are seen as defining the whole group, and the differences within the group and between individuals are overlooked. There is research to suggest that when people are stereotyped they will tend to live up to their stereotypical image. 'If that is what people say I am like, then that is what I will be like.'**

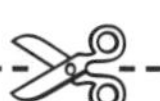

These questions guide you through the topic. If you need help to answer them, look at pages 222–225 of the Collins textbook.

11.5 short **questions** and **activities**

1. Using the information provided in this topic, identify six areas of inequality found in modern Britain.
2. Briefly describe two different forms of stratification.
3. Briefly describe how the kibbutzim in Israel attempted to create an unstratified society.
4. Describe the differences between the Registrar General's classification of occupations used in the 1991 Census and that used in 2001.
5. Explain the links between the concepts 'social exclusion' and the 'underclass'.
6. Describe the likely consequences for health and well-being of social exclusion.

summary worksheet

SOCIAL EXCLUSION

Joe and his friend Winston are both 20 years old. They have never managed to obtain paid work. Both grew up in an area of high unemployment. Joe and Winston's parents were all made redundant along with many of their neighbours when the local coalmine closed. They have been unable to find paid work since. There is over 30% unemployment on the estate where Joe and Winston live – and little chance of this improving. Because both of them stopped going to school regularly in Year 10, neither has any GCSEs. They didn't see the point at the time because there was no work or jobs for them to get anyway. Joe and Winston have a very negative view of the future and don't believe that they have any real opportunities in life. They have no training, they have never voted, they are not part of any organised community groups and admit that they are just drifting into the future with no plans, no ambitions and few prospects.

a Identify the areas of life in which Joe and Winston may be considered socially disadvantaged.

b Why might the Social Exclusion Unit regard Joe and Winston as members of the groups that they were set up to support?

c Drawing on previous learning and especially the work from Topics 1 and 4, describe how Joe and Winston's lifestyle might affect their physical, social, emotional and intellectual development.

d In which social class category would Joe, Winston and their families be registered in the 2001 Census?

e Identify three differences between the 2001 classification of class and the 1991 classification.

1

2

3

extension**activity**sheet

INEQUALITIES AND THE PROVISION OF CARE SERVICES

a Evaluate the statement presented at the beginning of this topic 'we are all middle class now'.

b Discuss the implications for the health and care services arising from the issues of inequality identified in this topic.

11.6 Poverty and welfare support

The issue of poverty is arguably a central theme within this unit, but it is a concept that is difficult to define – and therefore difficult to measure. This topic considers the sometimes competing definitions of poverty, the various attempts to measure the extent of poverty and government responses to the continuing issues of the poor. Before discussing the classic definitions of poverty and the associated studies of the poor, students, in the *Getting you thinking* section will consider their own definitions and views on what it is to be poor and, further, to consider what they see as the consequences of being poor in modern Britain.

Answers to the *Check your understanding* questions on page 229 of the Collins textbook.

1 **Primary and secondary poverty were terms introduced by Rowntree in the first of his famous studies of levels of poverty in the City of York. 'Primary poverty' referred to a level of income which was below that which would maintain physical health and efficiency. 'Secondary poverty' referred to a situation where a family's income would have been sufficient to maintain health and efficiency had they spent money only on essentials, i.e. the items on his list.**

2 **The benefit system, which has not changed significantly in structure since it was established in the years immediately after the Second World War, includes both means-tested and universal benefits. 'Universal benefits' refer to those monetary benefits paid to people in specific social circumstances regardless of their income. For example, people with children under the age of 16 are entitled to Child Benefit, regardless of their economic circumstances. This is to be contrasted with 'means-tested benefits' which are paid only to people whose total income and savings are below an agreed level, established by government, e.g. Income Support. These benefits are seen as a safety net to keep people from poverty and destitution. Students may point to the links with Rowntree's concept of the poverty line and the associated primary poverty.**

3 **Research would indicate that the groups in our society who are most vulnerable to poverty include older people, lone-parent families, the unemployed, people on low wages, and people with disabilities and chronic illnesses.**

4 **Reasons offered as to why there is a proportionately lower take-up of means-tested benefits than universal benefits may include:**
- **The complexity of the benefit system, especially for those benefits that are means-tested. People are often not clear of their entitlements. They may not even know the range of benefits that exist.**
- **The length and detail required in the forms that have to be completed.**
- **The perceived invasion into privacy. The questions are often seen as unnecessary and an unpleasant intrusion into personal circumstances.**
- **The view by some claimants that benefits are charity and not an entitlement. Some people, particularly older people, are too proud to claim their benefit, particularly the means-tested benefits.**
- **The perceived stigma attached to visiting benefit offices and claiming benefits at all.**

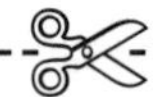

These questions guide you through the topic. If you need help to answer them, look at pages 226–229 of the Collins textbook.

11.6 short **questions** and **activities**

1 Why is 'poverty' difficult to define?

2 Explain the difference between absolute and relative poverty.

3 Who introduced the concept of the 'poverty line' and what does it mean?

4 Who introduced the concept of the 'culture of poverty' and what does it mean?

5 Briefly describe how the National Insurance scheme underpinned the benefit system set up following the Beveridge Report.

6 Briefly describe how Mack and Lansley in their 'Breadline Britain' studies measured levels of poverty.

summaryworksheet

THE TAKE-UP OF BENEFITS

Martha is 75 years of age. She lives on her state retirement pension and is finding it difficult to manage. An advice worker who visited the day centre she attends explained to Martha that she could also claim Income Support and additional housing benefit. Both of these are means-tested benefits. Martha became quite annoyed and impatient at this advice. She said 'I don't want the social prying into my private business. I haven't claimed anything in my life before and I'm not going to start now. Anyway it's so complicated. They want to know everything. And what if I get it wrong? I could be all over the newspapers if I claim too much.'

In the meantime, Martha is depressed and worried. She is frightened to put on the heating in the winter because she cannot afford the bills. Her diet is poor and her general quality of life declining.

a Referring to our definitions of absolute and relative poverty:

i Would you describe Martha as living in absolute or relative poverty?

....

ii Explain your answer

....

....

....

iii Compare your answers with other members of your group.

b Why is Martha reluctant to apply for Income Support and housing benefit?

....

....

....

c What are the likely consequences for Martha's health and well-being of not claiming these benefits?

....

....

....

d What measures could be taken to encourage people such as Martha to apply for benefits to which they are entitled?

....

....

UNIVERSAL AND MEANS-TESTED BENEFITS

a Using the internet, the library and other community resources (e.g. the Citizen's Advice Bureau), identify and briefly describe three means-tested and three universal benefits currently available.

b Discuss the view that 'universal benefits should be a thing of the past. All benefits should be for those in most financial need'.

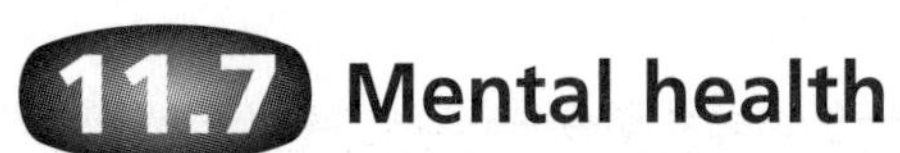

11.7 Mental health

Mental illness, like poverty, is also surrounded by difficulties of definition and measurement. The topic opens with a consideration of the difficulties of definition and the associated problems of measuring the prevalence of mental illness. There is a brief consideration of the possible causes of mental illness and the possible consequences of labelling a person as mentally ill. Finally there is discussion of the government response to the needs of the mentally ill and specifically the policy of care within the community rather than in large psychiatric hospitals.

The scenario provided in the *Getting you thinking* section will help students to focus on their own views and feelings about the much publicised issue of more routinely caring for the mentally ill in the community rather than in secure units or hospitals. They may benefit by taking brief notes during these discussions and returning to them when they have completed the topic and considering how far their views were supported by evidence.

Answers to the *Check your understanding* questions on page 233 of the Collins textbook.

1 **Mental illness is very common (and we will discuss the statistics that support this claim later in the section) but there is a great deal of controversy, discussion and uncertainty about what we mean by a mental illness, what are the causes and how people can be helped to recover. There are difficulties of definition. What is seen as normal and abnormal behaviour varies between societies and at different times in history. Further, there can be considerable difficulties in diagnosis and appropriate support when doctors, carers and clients are from different cultural or religious backgrounds.**

2 **The causes of mental illness and distress are not fully understood but are likely to be a consequence of both inherited characteristics (nature) and life experiences (nurture). It is likely that mental illness results from a range of factors including genetic or inherited characteristics, ongoing changes in our biochemistry (e.g. hormonal changes) and stressful life experiences (e.g. the consequences of divorce, bereavement or redundancy).**

Some students may add that it is possible that some people due to their genetic make-up are more vulnerable to mental illness than others which may be triggered by stressful or traumatic life events, e.g. divorce, redundancy or the death of a partner.

3 **'Institutionalisation' refers to the process of becoming dependent on the rules and routines of large organisations. Students may refer to the work of Erving Goffman who claimed that residents in large institutions (and he used mental hospitals as his main example) became so dependent on the rules and routines of these institutes that they were often unable to function independently in the 'outside' community.**

4 **The vast majority of people today with mental health problems are cared for within the community. Reasons for the movement towards community care for people with mental health problems include a view that it would be cheaper than running large hospitals. It has been seen, however, that this is not the case – good and effective community care is expensive. In terms of good practice it was held that large hospitals where not providing the appropriate care for the mentally ill and that they led to patients becoming dependent on the routines of the hospital that institutional care could lead to. Some students may refer to the fact that only a very small minority of mental health patients are a danger to themselves or others, and arguably do not need to be in a large protective environment like a hospital where 'normal' social life is suspended.**

5 **'Formal patients', who constitute approximately 15% of psychiatric patients in hospitals, are compulsorily detained under the Mental Health Act and lose some of the rights enjoyed by informal patients and other citizens. They cannot, by law, refuse treatment or leave the hospital. 'Informal patients', by contrast, are legally free to discharge themselves from hospital and they can refuse treatment. They have exactly the same rights as the people in hospital with physical ailments.**

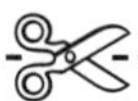

These questions guide you through the topic. If you need help to answer them, look at pages 230–233 of the Collins textbook.

11.7 short **questions** and **activities**

1 Why is it difficult to define the term 'mental illness'?

2 What is meant by the term 'labelling'? Identify one possible negative consequence of labelling.

3 How have the care services for people with mental illnesses changed during the past hundred years?

4 What is meant by the term 'multi-disciplinary team' in the context of care for the mentally ill?

5 Briefly describe the role of a Mental Health Review Tribunal.

6 Why is it difficult to accurately know the number of suicides in the UK?

summary worksheet

THE PREVALENCE OF MENTAL ILLNESS

Prevalence of mental health problems, by gender (people aged 16–64)

All figures are percentages

Diagnosis and rate (past week)	Female		Male		All	
	1993	2000	1993	2000	1993	2000
Mixed anxiety and depression	10.1	11.2	5.5	7.2	7.8	9.2
Generalised anxiety disorder	5.3	4.8	4.0	4.6	4.6	4.7
Depressive episode	2.8	3.0	1.9	2.6	2.3	2.8
Phobias	2.6	2.4	1.3	1.5	1.9	1.9
Obsessive–compulsive disorder	2.1	1.5	1.2	1.0	1.7	1.2
Panic disorder	1.0	0.7	0.9	0.8	1.0	0.7
Any neurotic disorder	19.9	20.2	12.6	14.4	16.3	17.3

Source: ONS, 2000, Psychiatric morbidity among adults living in private households in Great Britain.

Note: people may have more than one type of neurotic disorder, so the percentage with 'any neurotic disorder' is not the sum of those with specific disorders.

a What is meant by the term 'prevalence' used in the title of this table ? (You may need to refer to the KEY TERMS on page 106.)

b What is meant by the term 'morbidity 'in this context? (It may be helpful to refer to the KEY TERMS section on page 212.)

c According to the table, what was the prevalence of neurotic disorders in1993 and 2000?

d What does the table show about the difference between the mental health problems of men and women?

e Why is it difficult to measure accurately the prevalence of mental illness in the UK?

extension**activity**sheet

POLICY AND PRACTICE IN THE CARE OF THE MENTALLY ILL

a Evaluate how far the policy of community care has effectively met the needs of the mentally ill and their families.

b A public meeting has been called to discuss the opening of a residential unit for people with mental health problems in an urban neighbourhood. Working with a partner, prepare the arguments for and against this proposal in preparation for a debate on the issue.

11.8 Ability and disability

Disability is a term used in different ways by different writers, and the topic opens by considering this issue and its implication for policy-makers. There is then an associated discussion of the medical, psychological and social models of disability and the implications of each approach to policy and provision for people with disabilities. Finally there is a discussion of government responses to the needs of disabled people.

Getting you thinking will give students the opportunity to consider what it is they mean when they describe a person as disabled and to further consider the day-to-day impact of living with a physical disability. They can consider whether and how their school or college could be further adapted to meet the needs of people using wheelchairs.

Answers to the *Check your understanding* questions on page 237 of the Collins textbook.

1 **The Disability Discrimination Act defines disability as 'a physical or mental impairment that has a substantial and long-term adverse effect on a person's ability to carry out normal day-to-day activities'. Some students may explain that long-term normally means that the impairment has lasted or is likely to last for at least 12 months. Normal day-to-day activities includes things like eating, washing, walking and going shopping.**

2 **'Impairment' is a term used to describe the limitations or restrictions to day-to-day activities that are the result of a physical, mental or sensory dysfunction or illness. There is a focus on the individual's medical condition.**

3 **The medical model of disability refers to a view that regards disability as a dysfunction, an impairment or an illness located within the person's body. They have multiple sclerosis, for example, and the difficulties in day-to-day living would be seen as a consequence of their condition. The focus is on the individual patient. It would be seen as the individual's responsibility to adjust to the limitations to day-to-day life that may follow.**

The psychological model of disability also has its main focus on the individual with a particular concern that individuals should adjust to their condition. It will address the individual's mental response to their impairment and the therapy may be concerned with developing coping strategies.

The social model of disability, in contrast to the medical and psychological models, locates disability within society. The social model locates the problems not with the individual, but in the physical environment and in people's attitudes and practices. Students may refer to the 'disabling environment'. They may also give an example to illustrate their point, e.g. that the limitations on day-to-day activity for somebody in a wheelchair may be due to limited access to and within buildings, insufficient adaptation of public and domestic services and appliances and people's focus on their impairment with less interest in the range of their abilities.

4 **During the twentieth century people with disabilities may have become institutionalised because if they were not cared for at home by their family or friends, they were very likely to have been cared for in hospitals and other institutions. Many of these were large institutions, some of them one-time workhouses, largely separated from the wider society. 'Patients' were cared for by medical, nursing and other care staff and the institutions were managed like hospital wards, with the associated rules, routines and procedures. The danger and concern was that 'patients' would became so dependent on the rules and routines of these institutes that they would be unable to function independently in the community. They would become institutionalised.**

5 **In answering this question students may draw from Topic 3 (The ageing society) and specifically the section concerned with the care of the vulnerable elderly.**

The NHS Community Care Act 1990 was key to the development and delivery of care services outside institutions and within communities. It required local authorities to:

(i) Assess the needs of people requesting community care services. Students may also add that the 1995 Carers (Recognition of Services) Act gave informal carers the right to a separate assessment of their needs too.
(ii) Manage the provision of community care services across the community.
(iii) Appoint, in complex cases, a care manager to plan, monitor and review the provision for users and their carers.
(iv) Purchase services for their clients from statutory, private and voluntary providers. The care may include home care services, meals on wheels, attendance at a day centre or lunch club, adaptations to their own home, or full-time care in a residential care home.

Students may refer to the more recent 1996 Community Care (Direct Payments) Act which took this policy further – following assessment, disabled people may receive cash payments from the local authority to buy their own care services rather than have the arrangements made for them.

6 **In answering this question students may draw from Topic 4 (Discrimination and access to health and care services) where the Disability Discrimination Act 1995 is discussed in more detail. The areas of economic and social life covered by the act are:**

(i) Employment, where
- **it is unlawful to treat a person less favourably (without justification) than other employees or job applicants because of his or her disability**
- **it is required that employers make reasonable adjustments to the working environment to meet the needs of people with disabilities.**

(ii) Access to goods, facilities and services, where
- **it is unlawful to treat a person less favourably because they are disabled**
- **service providers have to consider making reasonable adjustments to the way they deliver their services so that people can use them.**
- **service providers have to consider making permanent physical adjustments to their premises.**

(iii) buying or renting land or property.

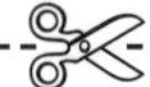

These questions guide you through the topic. If you need help to answer them, look at pages 234–237 of the Collins textbook.

11.8 short **questions** and **activities**

1 Why is it difficult to define the term disability?

2 Why is it difficult to measure the prevalence of disability in our society?

3 Why may it be helpful to make a distinction between the terms 'impairment' and 'disability'?

4 Explain the differences between the three models of disability discussed in this topic.

5 How have the care services for people with disabilities changed during the past hundred years?

6 What change to the management of care provision was introduced by the Community Care (Direct Payments) Act 1996?

summary worksheet

CARE SERVICES FOR PEOPLE WITH DISABILITIES

Mohammed is 61 and has Parkinson's Disease. Tamsila, his wife, is his main carer. Because she has arthritis, Tamsila is not very strong, finds walking painful and so she doesn't get out much. Tamsila feels pessimistic about the future and is quite depressed. Neither Mohammed nor Tamsila speak very much English and they feel quite socially isolated.

Mohammed needs considerable help with daily living activities. He and his wife have recently been assessed by the local social services department for a range of community care services. They are going to receive a direct payment for these services so that they can chose their own care providers and pay them directly. Tamsila would like to use people from the mosque, who she knows and with whom she feels comfortable.

a Define the term 'impairment'.

b Describe how Mohammed and his wife are physically impaired.

c How might a care professional using the psychological approach to disability address their issues and concerns?

d How might a care professional using the social model of disability approach the issues?

e What are the possible advantages and disadvantages to the family of direct payments in the provision of their care services?

Advantages

Disadvantages

extension**activity**sheet

DISABILITY POLICY AND PRACTICE

a Discuss the view that, despite legislation, we still live in a 'disabling environment'.

b Evaluate how effective government measures have been in meeting the care needs of people with disabilities.

c Compare and contrast the three models of disability introduced in this topic and evaluate their contribution to the care of people with disabilities.

Understanding Human Behaviour is an externally tested unit and will require students to answer questions on aspects of all the different care settings: health, early years (care and education), care of older people and individuals with specific needs. Students will be expected to demonstrate knowledge and understanding of the material in the specification. They will also be expected to apply their knowledge and understanding to unfamiliar situations. In addition, there will be opportunities for the students to demonstrate their research and analytical skills and also to make evaluations of material presented to them. Students should have an understanding of the different influences on behaviour and their effects. They should also know about different theoretical approaches that help care workers to understand human behaviour, and how they are applied in health and social care contexts. They should understand the principles of each approach and the advantages and disadvantages of using the approaches in different situations. Many of the questions will relate to real-life case studies, and practice in answering questions relating to case studies will help students prepare well for the examination.

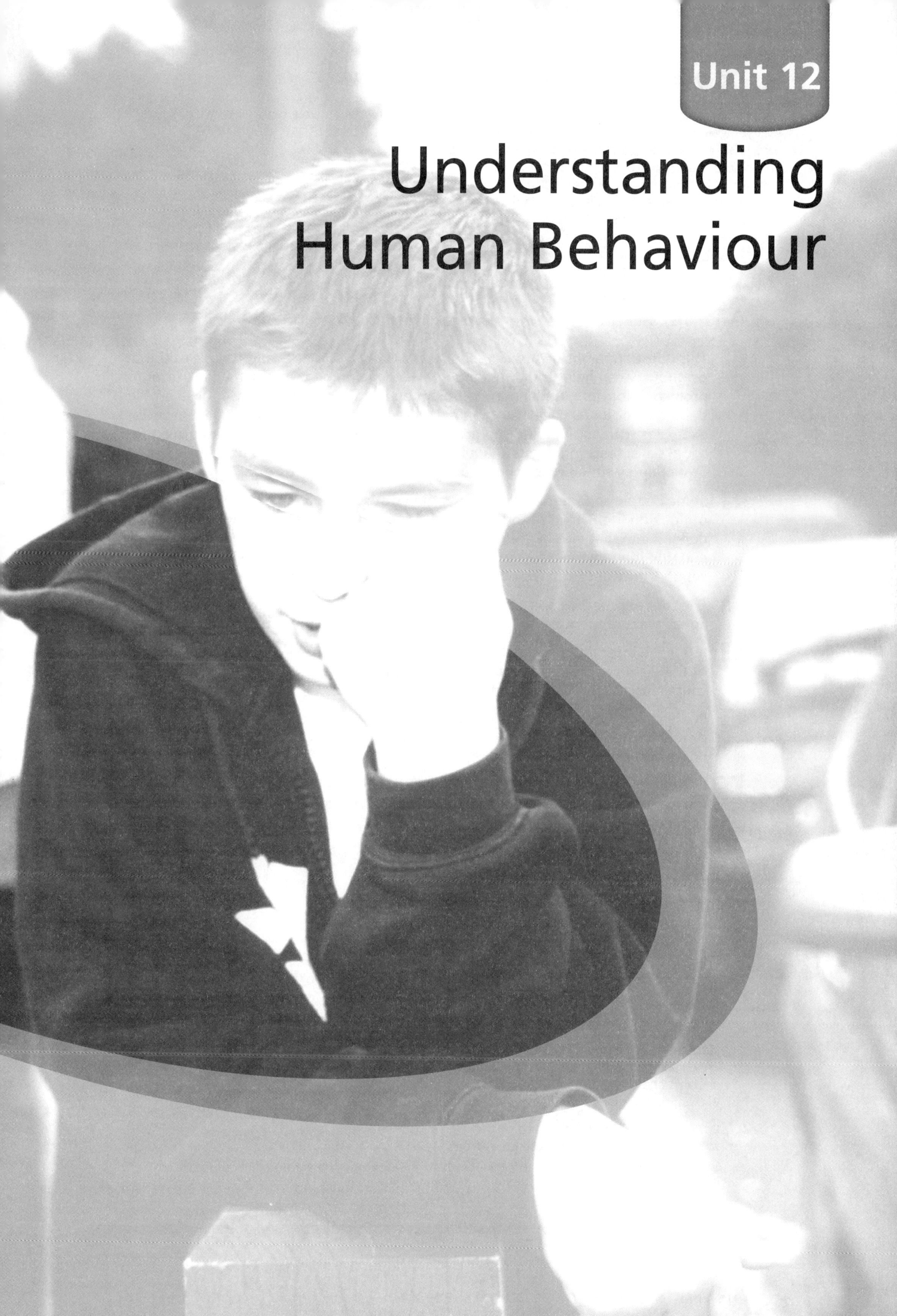

Unit 12

Understanding Human Behaviour

12.1 Using psychology in care work

This topic introduces some of the ways in which psychology can help care practitioners in their work. It looks at the different ways in which people feel about themselves, especially when they are ill. Students are asked to consider what constitutes problem behaviour – and for whom is it a problem. There are many psychological and developmental problems and we see some ways in which they are classified. Students are introduced to the idea of counselling which is developed further in Topics 5, 6 and 7. As this unit is about psychology and care work, students are also introduced to the idea that the behaviour of care practitioners is important, and this is linked to the care value base.

The *Getting you thinking* activities are designed to get students thinking about how a knowledge of psychology might help care practitioners in their work with a variety of service users. It is easier to think about this if there are specific examples to discuss. A starting point might be to get the students to identify the problems in each example and the care practitioners that would be involved.

Answers to the *Check your understanding* questions on page 245 of the Collins textbook.

1 **This question might be answered in several ways. Students might have said that psychology can help us understand normal development and behaviour, recognise problem behaviour, understand problem behaviour, classify and diagnose problem behaviour or understand our own behaviour. Students might have given specific examples such as changing the behaviour of a child with autism to improve their social skills, teaching a young adult with learning disabilities to use public transport, or working with an older person who is unhappy of depressed.**

2 **Some people cope better with illness than others mainly because of their positive outlook on life. They see the glass as 'half full' instead of 'half empty'. It might also depend on what else in going on in their lives, what they know about the illness and whether anyone they know has had the illness. It could also depend on the support they get from their family and friends.**

3 **The four approaches are: statistical; deviation from social norms; deviation of an 'ideal' state of mental health; and whether people are able to function adequately.**

4 **ICD is the international classification of diseases. The DSM-IV is the fourth revision of the diagnostic and statistical manual of the American Psychiatric Association, containing nearly 300 categories of mental disorder.**

5 **People might seek help from a counsellor if they have problems with their marriage or relationships, post-traumatic stress after a serious incident in their lives, or if they misuse drugs or alcohol.**

6 **Practitioners should examine their own behaviour as it affects the way in which they provide care for their clients. For example, do they listen actively and communicate well?**

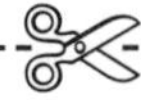

These questions guide you through the topic. If you need help to answer them, look at pages 240–245 of the Collins textbook.

12.1 short **questions** and **activities**

1. Look at the seven statements about thinking and feeling which illustrate where psychology can help in care work. For each statement, write down the age ranges to which you think it applies. Compare your answers and the reasons for your answers with someone else's.
2. List two practitioners from each of the following areas who might use ideas from psychology in their work: health, social work and education.
3. What five questions are important in deciding whether or not we are 'ill'?
4. What three factors are thought to contribute to someone taking or not taking their medication?
5. List the three main categories of mental disorder, according to the DSM-IV.
6. List the four main approaches to counselling, and identify some of the people who train to become counsellors.
7. Explain what is meant by the phrase 'care practitioners' behaviour'.

THINKING POSITIVELY

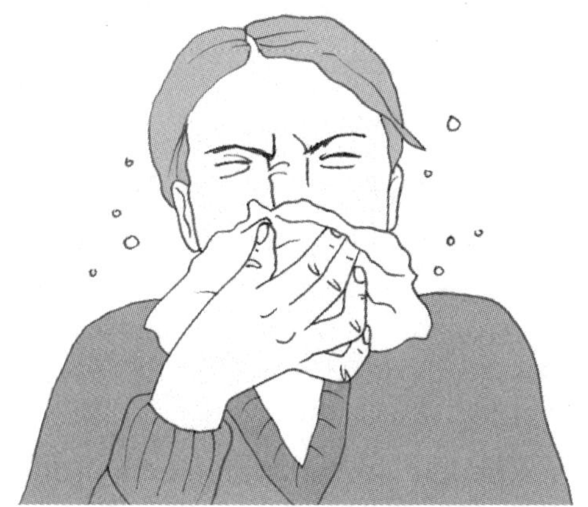

a Complete the table by placing a tick in the appropriate box, against each of the statements.

Statement	Positive attitude	Negative attitude
It's just a tickly cough.		
I am going to go to work.		
I need some medicine.		
It must be a virus.		
I'll be better by the weekend.		
I need to be better to go to the party at the weekend.		
It might last for weeks.		
I just need a bit of a rest.		

b Explain the following sentence, ' Kate always sees her glass as half empty, whereas Emma always sees her glass as half full'.

....

....

....

extension**activity**sheet

PROBLEM BEHAVIOUR – BUT WHOSE PROBLEM?

a Read the section on problem behaviour (pages 242–243), including the case study.

- **i** Who is Maggie's incontinence a problem to?
- **ii** Imagine you are the manager of the care home. What advice would you give to Jenny?

b Describe some other behaviours that might be seen in a residential care home that could be regarded as problem behaviours. For each of these behaviours, explain who it might be a problem for.

c Work in pairs for this activity. Take a walk around your school or college or around the area you live.

- **i** List some of the things you see people do that would be a problem to someone. Say who you think they are a problem to.
- **ii** Give a reason for including each of the items in your list.
- **iii** Compare your list and reasons with your partner's. Note down where you and your partner disagree.
- **iv** Share your findings with the rest of the class and discuss them.

12.2 Factors affecting our behaviour

Students will be familiar with the idea that our characteristics are determined by genetic and environmental factors. They may not be so familiar with the complexity of this, the fact that most behaviour we show is a result of many of these factors. This topic focuses on a wide range of 'environmental' factors, and considers in detail some psychological factors and sociological factors. The importance of early attachment is discussed and it is important for students to realise that not everyone shares the same view and that practitioners' views have changed over time. The importance of later experiences is discussed, as well as that of early experiences.

The case study in the *Getting you thinking* section is a situation that will be familiar to most students. However, how many of them will have asked these particular questions? This is likely to spark off an interesting discussion.

Answers to the *Check your understanding* questions on page 251 of the Collins textbook.

1 **Most practitioners focus on the influences that come from people's environment rather than on those that come from their genetic make-up, because the latter cannot be changed. Environmental influences, such as the experiences their service users will have, may be altered.**

2 **A psychologist would be interested in the experiences of the service users as individuals, such as their early experiences, early socialisation and other things that happen to them within their lives. A sociologist would be interested in the sort of influences that arise because of service users' membership of certain groups within society, e.g. gender, social class and ethnic groups.**

3 **Students might have said: attachment to a parent or carer; early experiences are important for emotional development; or evidence on bonding is contradictory.**

4 **Early experiences provide stimulation and models to help children communicate. Play gives opportunities for a child's environment to be explored. This means they develop thinking skills.**

5 **Following bereavement, a person goes through shock and disbelief, then a longing for the person who has died, and perhaps denial. This leads to a period of deep sadness and, finally, the pain and sadness will start to fade.**

These questions guide you through the topic. If you need help to answer them, look at pages 246–251 of the Collins textbook.

12.2 short **questions** and **activities**

1. Explain what is meant by 'nature–nurture' influences on our lives.
2. Give two examples of genetic factors and two examples of environmental influences.
3. Define what is meant by 'cognitive' development.
4. Explain how children who have 'missed out' in earlier years may still progress well.
5. Read the case study about Jemma (page 249). Explain how she has been affected by bullying or unfair discrimination.
6. List the different ways, other than gender, age and ethnic group, that sociologists might group people.
7. Explain what the most important experiences are that care practitioners can offer to their service users.

12.2 **summary** worksheet

NATURE, NURTURE OR BOTH?

Here is a list of factors that determine the way we are. Some of our characteristics are determined by our genes alone, some by our environment alone, and some by both our genes and our environment.

- Gender
- Having the condition cystic fibrosis
- Weight
- Colour of hair
- Colour of eyes
- Having influenza
- Strength
- Being depressed
- Having no friends.

a Place a letter 'G' after those you believe are determined by genes alone.

b Place a letter 'B' after those you believe are determined by both genes and by the environment.

c List any that you have not placed a letter against. If you have placed a letter beside all of them, explain why.

....

....

....

d Explain what type of factor influences children's language development.

....

....

THE IMPORTANCE OF EARLY ATTACHMENTS AND EXPERIENCES

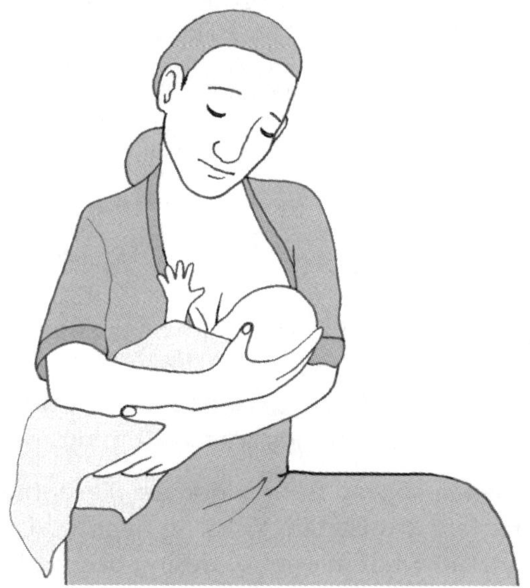

a Some people believe that early attachments are important for successful development.

i Summarise, in your own words, the evidence that early attachments are crucial for successful development.

ii Outline the evidence that suggests otherwise.

b Find out about 'Sure Start'. Summarise your findings under these headings:

i Who is responsible for the programme?

ii What are the aims of the programme?

iii What type of people work as part of the programme?

iv How does the programme work?

v What has the programme achieved so far?

12.3 Theories of behaviour and a problem-solving framework

This topic introduces students to the idea of a theory and the reasons why theoretical knowledge is helpful to care practitioners. Students learn about a problem-solving framework and how theoretical knowledge can be used in practice. This is useful for getting students to understand how a mental health worker goes about their work. The benefits and drawbacks of diagnosis and labelling of conditions is discussed. Sensitivity should be employed when discussing these issues, as some students or members of their families may have a diagnosed condition.

Getting you thinking is designed to get students to discuss how the advice given by a layperson with experience of the world might differ from that given by various health care professionals. It should get them to think about how the advice given by health care professionals working in different fields might vary according to their expertise. The students might also like to consider what advice a grandmother might be able to give that a health care professional might not.

Answers to the *Check your understanding* questions on page 257 of the Collins textbook.

1 **Theories can help care practitioners understand the behaviour of a service user. Some theories may also help in solving problems. They may help care practitioners understand why something has happened and what has gone wrong. They may also help them when they try to put things right.**

2 **The four stages of the problem-solving framework are: Assessment, where information about the problem is collected, Working hypothesis where an attempt is made to understand what might be causing or contributing to the problem, Intervention where a change may be made to make things better, and Review where a decision is made whether or not the intervention has been successful. It is a cycle, as the process may be ongoing, with another assessment coming after the review.**

3 **A diagnosis is important in helping people who have problems as it gives them a way to understand their problems and explain them to other people. It also suggests where they may look to find out more for themselves, or link up with local support groups and other voluntary organisations.**

4 **Some people think that a diagnosis is not helpful because for some conditions there is no clear view amongst experts about what the condition actually is. Sometimes there is no treatment, so why have a diagnosis? Sometimes it is just a way of describing someone's behaviour without actually adding anything to our understanding of it. It could be seen as labelling people, which could lead to people being stereotyped and not seen as individuals in their own right.**

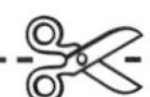

These questions guide you through the topic. If you need help to answer them, look at pages 252–257 of the Collins textbook.

12.3 short **questions** and **activities**

1. Describe what is meant by 'common sense' and explain how this differs from a 'theory'.
2. List four of the main approaches to understanding behaviour.
3. Make up a table that shows the different stages in the problem-solving framework, and for each stage give two aspects that might be involved.
4. What would a psychologist do if a review showed that the intervention had not worked?
5. Describe how psychological theories may be linked to practice in the problem-solving framework cycle.
6. Explain why it is more difficult to diagnose autism than it is to diagnose diabetes.

summary worksheet

APPLYING THE PROBLEM-SOLVING FRAMEWORK

This diagram shows the stages of the problem-solving framework. It may even be applied to situations that do not require using a psychological theory.

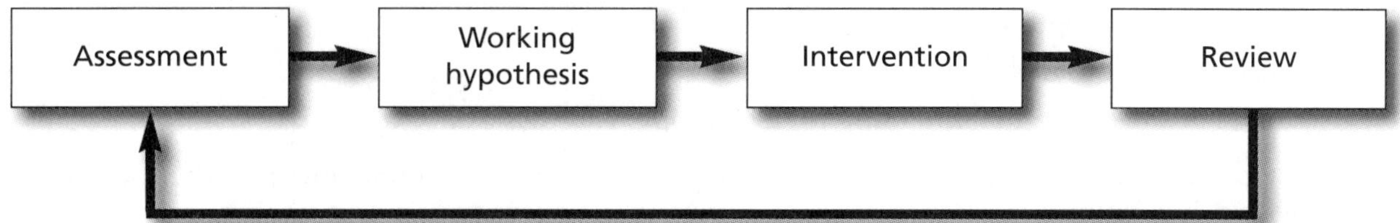

Read this case study and answer the questions that follow.

Lee is three years old and wets the bed most nights. His mother, Tracey, says that this has been happening for over a year, and she is fed up having to wash his sheets every day. She asks her friend, Lisa, who has had four children what she could do to stop him wetting the bed. Lisa asks Tracey how much Lee has to drink before he goes to bed. Tracey says that he only has three drinks between tea and bedtime. Lisa suggests that Tracey only allows Lee to have one drink, at the most, between tea and bedtime. She thinks that if he drinks less, then his bladder will not get so full and therefore he will not wet the bed. Tracey says she will try this, and get back to Lisa in three weeks to let her know if this has made a difference. After three weeks, Tracey meets Lisa and tells her that it has been difficult to get Lee to drink less and anyway she has not seen much difference in the frequency of the bed-wetting. Lisa suggests that if it is difficult to get Lee to drink less, Tracey should wake Lee up when she goes to bed and take him to the toilet. This should mean that his bladder is less full.

a Identify what is happening in the four stages of the problem-solving framework in the case study.

i assessment ....

....

ii working hypothesis ....

....

iii intervention ....

....

iv review ....

....

b Explain how the outcome of the review results in Tracey and Lisa going round the cycle again.

....

....

extension**activity**sheet

TO DIAGNOSE OR NOT?

Find out about a condition called dyslexia.

a Write a paragraph about dyslexia under the following headings:

- Some of the symptoms
- How easy it is to diagnose
- Some of the things that are done to help people with dyslexia.

b Some people believe that diagnosing and naming conditions is helpful, whereas other people believe it is unhelpful.

i Give two reasons why diagnosing someone as dyslexic may be helpful to them.

1 ....

....

....

2 ....

....

....

ii Give two reasons why diagnosing someone as dyslexic may not be helpful to them.

1 ....

....

....

2 ....

....

....

12.4 Behavioural approaches

Behavioural approaches are very important and effective. Students should be encouraged to understand why behaviour should be described as precisely as possible. They should know about the different ways behaviour may be reinforced. There can sometimes be misconceptions about the nature of negative reinforcement as it can be confused with punishment. There are various terms associated with behavioural approaches that students need to know and understand, such as shaping behaviour, time out, token economies and vicarious reinforcement. An understanding of these could be important for gaining high marks in the examination.

The case study in the *Getting you thinking* section sets the scene for the topic and invites students to voice their opinions at the start. The case study is revisited towards the end of the topic when the ABC approach is discussed. This is a chance to consolidate students' understanding of the problem-solving framework by applying it to this case study. The students could then revisit the initial question and see how much more detailed and specific their answer would be, having studied the topic.

Answers to the *Check your understanding* questions on page 263 of the Collins textbook.

1 **Reinforcement is a 'reward' of some kind, and behaviour which is reinforced or rewarded is likely to be repeated. Positive reinforcement happens when something pleasant occurs. Negative reinforcement occurs when something unpleasant stops.**

2 **Punishment is different from negative reinforcement. Punishment is when something unpleasant starts to happen, whereas negative reinforcement is when something unpleasant stops happening.**

3 **'Shaping' behaviour is used when a service user cannot actually perform the behaviour that the care practitioner wants to encourage. 'Shaping' is when behaviour near to that wanted is looked for and reinforced. An example would be someone who is frightened of planes being able to go to an airport to see planes taking off without actually going on one.**

4 **Vicarious reinforcement is indirect reinforcement. An example would be seeing someone being rewarded for doing something, then showing the same behaviour ourselves.**

5 **A token economy is where something of no real value, like stars, is given for appropriate behaviour. A reward may be given when enough 'stars' have been collected.**

6 **'A' stands for antecedent, e.g. what happens just before a particular behaviour occurs. 'B' stands for behaviour – what the person actually does. 'C' stands for consequences – what happens after the behaviour occurs.**

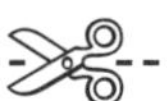

These questions guide you through the topic. If you need help to answer them, look at pages 258–263 of the Collins textbook.

12.4 short **questions** and **activities**

1 Give the three propositions of a behavioural approach.

2 Why is it important to be as specific as possible when describing behaviour?

3 Give two examples of the way in which positive reinforcement may change behaviour.

4 Explain how a particular behaviour may be extinguished by ignoring it.

5 Explain the difference between continuous reinforcement and intermittent reinforcement.

6 Re-write the seven features of a behavioural approach in your own words.

DIFFERENT TYPES OF REINFORCEMENT

a There are different ways of influencing behaviour – positive reinforcement, negative reinforcement and punishment. The drawing below shows one such way of reinforcing behaviour.

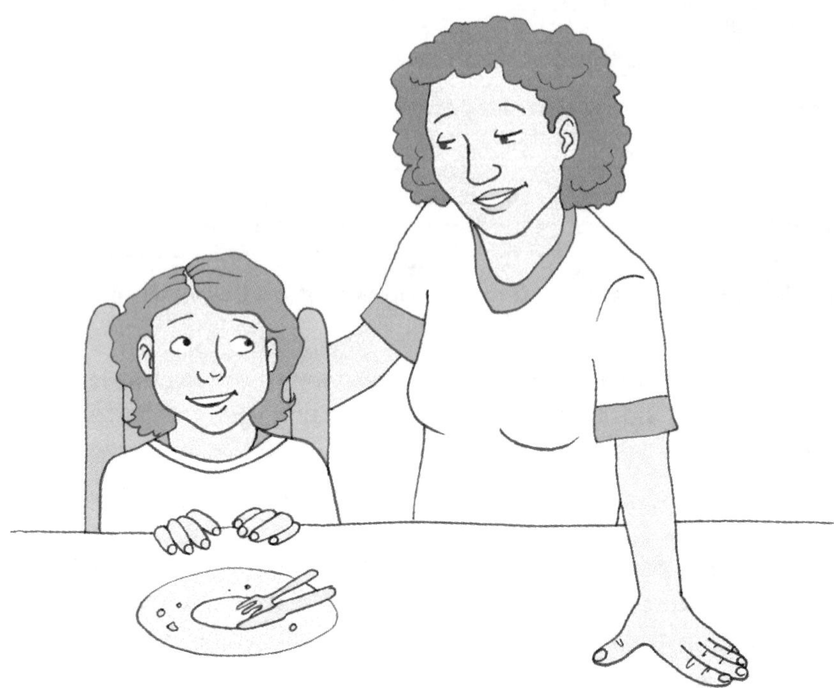

i What type of reinforcement is shown in the drawing?

....

ii What is the child likely to do when she has her next meal?

....

....

b Complete the table by ticking the correct box alongside each example of behaviour reinforcement.

Behaviour	*Positive reinforcement*	*Negative reinforcement*	*Punishment*
Teenager studies hard for his exams; gets a new bike from his parents.			
Middle-aged man stops smoking; no longer breathless when climbing stairs.			
Child tidies her room; praised by her parents.			
Child hits his sister; not allowed to watch TV.			
Student gets her coursework completed; teacher stops nagging.			
Children play well together; father takes them to the park.			

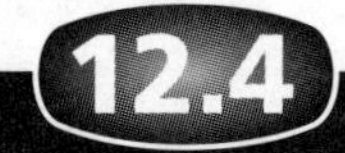

extension**activity**sheet

THE ABC OF THE BEHAVIOURAL APPROACH

Read the section about the ABC approach to assessment on page 261.

a Design a table that summarises the main points of each part of the ABC approach to assessment.

b Add another column to your table that describes how the ABC approach to assessment is used in the case study in which Lorna uses a behavioural approach to change Jamie's behaviour (page 262).

c Construct a flow chart, using the problem-solving framework you met in the previous topic, to tell the story of how Lorna manages to change Jamie's behaviour. Try to use as few words as possible, yet still get across the main points.

12.5 Cognitive approaches

In this topic the students are introduced to the cognitive approach to understanding behaviour and to cognitive behaviour therapy, as the form of counselling which is based on it. Students should find the basic ideas easy to follow, although some of the terms used may seem confusing at first. The cognitive approach, like the behavioural approach, uses an ABC model to explain behaviour, but the letters refer to something quite different. Students need to understand these differences but will have achieved a good grounding in both theories when they do.

The case study in the *Getting you thinking* section is one that most students will be able to relate to. They may have experienced something like this themselves or know someone else who has. Sensitivity should be used during discussions in case there is someone who may be feeling vulnerable because of being involved in a similar situation. Students should be able to come up with similar situations and this is a good lead into a discussion about rational and distorted thinking.

Answers to the *Check your understanding* questions on page 269 of the Collins textbook.

1 **A cognitive approach is so-called because 'cognitive' means to do with thinking, and such an approach focuses on what a person is thinking.**

2 **The cognitive approach places a stress on what we think and believe because this affects what we feel and do. In cognitive behavioural therapy, we help people to examine their beliefs and to adopt new beliefs – so that they feel and act differently.**

3 **Examples might include thinking that someone doesn't like you because they haven't phoned and thinking that they prefer someone else. You might think this because you are feeling insecure. Another example might be if your friend is in a bad mood and you believe that you must have upset them. This might arise if you think you have said something that they might not approve of.**

4 **A dysfunctional belief is one that is faulty and not helpful to us.**

5 **In cognitive therapy, 'A' is the activating event, 'B' refers to the beliefs a person has about this activating event, and 'C stands for the consequences (behavioural or emotional).**

6 **Clients are asked to do homework because it keeps them involved between sessions. It will keep them focused on any new belief that is being trialled. It also provides the information about the intervention to be reviewed at the next meeting.**

7 **When working with clients who are depressed, the therapist should be aware that their thinking could be very negative and that they might find it difficult to commit to making any changes. They should be aware that any small positive change could be crucial in breaking the cycle of depression.**

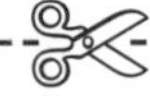

These questions guide you through the topic. If you need help to answer them, look at pages 264–269 of the Collins textbook.

12.5 short questions and activities

1 Identify three 'things' that go on inside people's heads.

2 What comes between the stimulus and the response, according to the cognitive approach?

3 Explain, in your own words, what 'cognitive primacy' means.

4 Make a flow chart to show how dysfunctional beliefs may arise.

5 Re-write in your own words, the four special challenges when using a cognitive approach with people who are depressed.

summary worksheet

ABC (BEHAVIOURAL) AND ABC (COGNITIVE)

There are two different ABC models of assessment, one when using a behavioural approach and another when using a cognitive approach.

a Complete the table to show what A, B and C refer to in each approach.

Stages	*Behavioural approach*	*Cognitive approach*
A		
B		
C		

b Looking now at the cognitive approach, think of an example which illustrates the ABC (cognitive) approach to assessment.

....

....

....

....

....

APPLYING THE ABC OF THE COGNITIVE APPROACH

a Re-read the case study about the ABC approach and how it is applied to John (pages 266–268). Make sure you can identify activating events, beliefs and consequences.

b Read the case study below and write a short account of how a cognitive approach might be used, explaining the reasons behind your suggestions.

> Sandra is 15 and attends her local secondary school. She lives out of town and has to catch a bus. She is a partially hearing and thinks that she is overweight. She says that she has no friends and that no one likes her. Recently, she has started to play truant. She says there is no point in going to school. She has agreed to meet with a counsellor.

c Write a similar case study of your own.

- **i** Explain why you think a cognitive approach might work in your case study.
- **ii** Give the case study to another member of the class (without them seeing your explanations) and ask them to write a short account of how a cognitive approach might be used, explaining the reasons behind their suggestions.
- **iii** Discuss with the other person any differences between their account and explanations and your own.

12.6 Pyschodynamic approaches

Many students may well be familiar with some of the ideas in this topic. They might have heard of Freud, and will almost certainly have heard of pyschoanalysis. They should find the idea of the id, ego and superego interesting, but it may take some time for them to sort out the differences between them. There are case studies that illustrate the use of psychoanalysis, and the students will need to work through these carefully. The summary worksheet provides a good focus and should reinforce their understanding.

The *Getting you thinking* section will get the students to focus on themselves and how it is sometimes difficult to explain why we think and act as we do. It may be useful to provide some specific examples, if the students find this activity difficult. These examples could be drawn from everyday situations, such as feeling angry or sad or happy. Are there always obvious reasons for feeling in this way? Is there some underlying issue in the past that influences this?

Answers to the *Check your understanding* questions on page 275 of the Collins textbook.

1

	Id	**Ego**	**Superego**
Conscious?	No	*Yes*	Yes
Concerned with?	*Immediate satisfaction*	*Allows us to cope with the demands of life*	Conscience and moral values
Operates according to?	*Pleasure principle*	Reality principle	*Perfection principle*
If it is not controlled, will lead to what?	Instinctive and immoral behaviour	The ego operates as the controlling system	*Overly moral behaviour*

2 **A psychoanalysist might explore a person's unconscious by: simply listening and interpreting what they say; using free association; interpreting dreams; hypnosis; interpreting play or drawings. In each case, what the person says or does has to be interpreted, not taken at face value.**

3 **In transactional analysis a stroke refers to recognition, such as a 'hug' or 'praise'. A game occurs when 'strokes' are interchanged. Things may not always be what they seem, such as a person appearing interested when in reality they are not.**

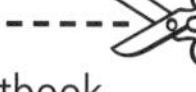

These questions guide you through the topic. If you need help to answer them, look at pages 270–275 of the Collins textbook.

12.6 short **questions** and **activities**

1. Who is considered responsible for the introduction of 'psychoanalysis'? What century was this? Where did he live?
2. Describe in as few words as you can, the difference between 'conscious' and 'unconscious'.
3. What do all ego defence mechanisms have in common?
4. Why might it be difficult for a pyschotherapist to find out what is happening in a person's unconscious?
5. Give two ways in which Bowlby's work has influenced care practice.
6. What is meant by a 'transaction'? What needs to happen before we can understand what a 'transaction' really means?

12.6 summary worksheet

GETTING TO THE UNCONSCIOUS

You will need to refer to the case study about Sasha (page 273) to answer these questions.

a The educational psychologist used a behavioural approach with Sasha. Identify the:

Antecedents ....

....

Behaviour ....

....

Consequences ....

....

b The psychotherapist explores some of Sasha's unconscious thoughts.

i Explain why the method of 'free-association' does not work very well with Sasha.

....

....

ii What two approaches work best with Sasha?

1 ....

2 ....

iii What hypothesis does the psychotherapist now have about Sasha's behaviour?

....

....

iv Identify the common thread in what Sasha says and does and what the psychotherapist thinks.

....

....

....

GETTING DEEPER INTO PSYCHOTHERAPY

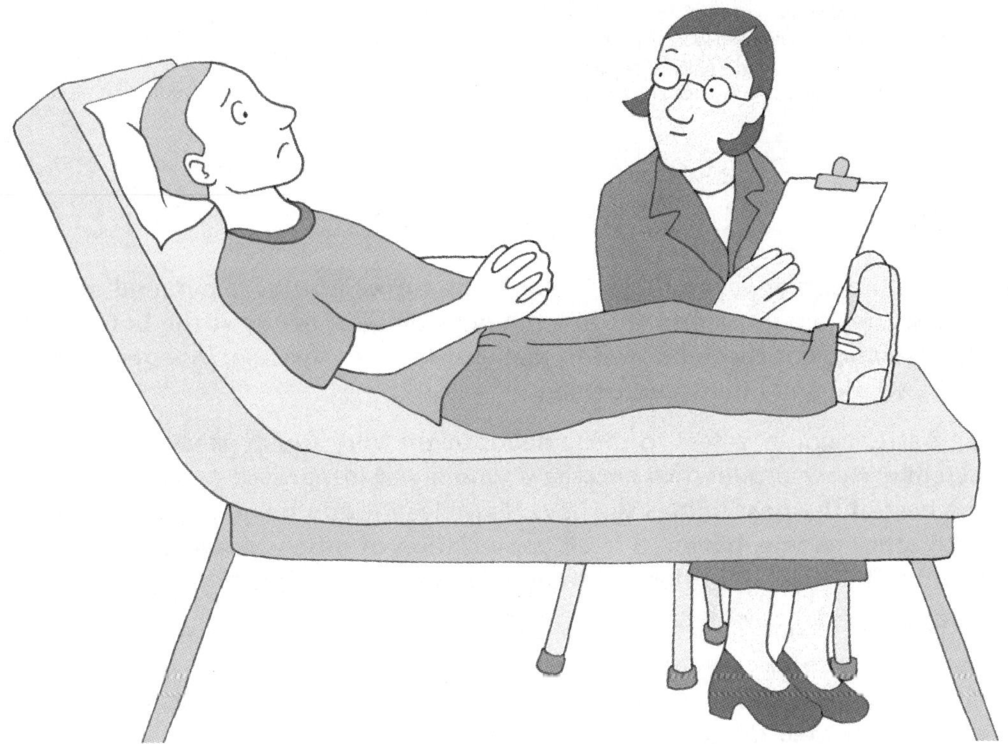

a Construct a table that compares the four common ego defence mechanisms in Freud's theory. You should have three headings: name of defence mechanism; simple description of the mechanism; an example of the mechanism.

b Read the following case study and answer the questions that follow.

> Robbie is 28 and lives on his own now. His partner, Rose, has just left him and said it was because Robbie never wanted to take her out anywhere. All he wanted to do was to play on his playstation every evening. Robbie misses Rose and wants her back. He says he finds it difficult to talk to people and he gets upset easily. Rose says that she is not coming back until he gets help. Robbie agrees to visit a psychotherapist.

i Imagine you are the psychotherapist. Outline the procedures that you might adopt with Robbie, giving reasons for your choices.

ii Suggest how an understanding of transactional analysis might help Rose and Robbie's relationship.

12.7 Humanistic approaches

Humanistic (person-centred) approaches are not the easiest to understand. The topic starts with Maslow's hierarchy of needs, which is something concrete for the students to get their teeth into. It then looks at the difficult ideas of 'self'. The core conditions of person-centred therapy are highlighted and what actually happens in person-cented counselling is discussed. Students may well think that this is not really counselling at all, as nothing much seems to be happening much of the time. The topic ends by seeing how this type of couselling forms the basis of what we know as the care value base.

The *Getting you thinking* section highlights one of the main aspects of the humanistic (person-centred) approach, as it gets the students to see the importance of empathy in this type of approach.

Answers to the *Check your understanding* questions on page 281 of the Collins textbook.

1 **'Higher-order' needs are those towards the top of Maslow's pyramid of needs. They are not a priority, like the physiological needs at the bottom of the pyramid, but those needed to make us feel worthwhile, independent and a whole and integrated person.**

2 **'Self-actualisation' refers to those needs at the very top of Maslow's pyramid, those required to become a whole and integrated person, making the best of the possibilities we have. Exmples include being able to identify with other people, having a fresh appreciation of other people and being creative. Maslow identified Beethoven and Abraham Lincoln.**

3 **A therapist is 'non-directive' when he or she allows the client the opportunity to discuss difficult feelings and experiences within a trusting environment, without asking particular questions. The client sets the direction of their discussions.**

4 **Core conditions are: unconditional positive regard for the client, empathy (stepping into the client's shoes) and genuineness (with the counsellor being felt to be 'real' person).**

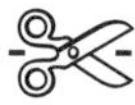

These questions guide you through the topic. If you need help to answer them, look at pages 276–281 of the Collins textbook.

12.7 short **questions** and **activities**

1. Make a table that names Maslow's six levels of needs, with a brief description of each need in your own words.
2. Write a short paragraph describing the features a person would have if they were 'self-actualising'. Do you know such a person?
3. There are a lot of 'selfs' in humanistic psychology. Make a list of them and explain what each means.
4. Explain the differerence, as simply as you can, between an internal locus of control and an external locus of control. How do these relate to the work of a humanistic counsellor?
5. What is the main difference between person-centred therapy and other methods of therapy? What is the most important feature of person-centred therapy?
6. Give some examples of non-verbal signals a counsellor might use to show empathy with a client.
7. What four things does person-centred counselling give a client the chance to do?

ORDER OF NEEDS

Here are Maslow's level of needs, but they are not in order.

- Belongingness
- Self-esteem needs
- Safety needs
- Self-actualisation needs
- Physiological needs
- Love needs

a Put the level of needs in the correct order, starting with the most basic.

1 ....

2 ....

3 ....

4 ....

5 ....

6 ....

b Which level of needs matches up with these descriptions?

i We need to avoid pain and harm.

....

ii We need to feel that we are worthwhile people.

....

iii We need air, water and food, and some degree of physical comfort.

....

c What is meant by saying that the way in which we grow and develop is an active process?

....

....

....

extension**activity**sheet

USING A HUMANISTIC (PERSON-CENTRED) COUNSELLING APPROACH IN A CARE SETTING

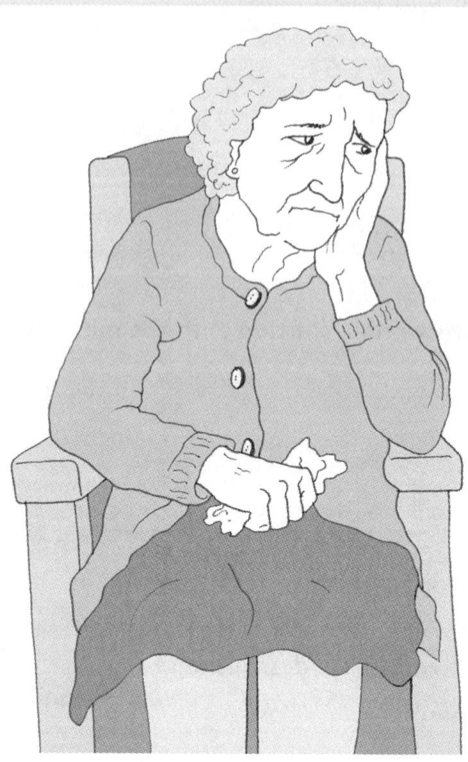

Read the following case study and answer the questions that follow.

Mary is 84 and is in residential care. Her husband died about a month ago and she just sits in a chair all day and says very little. She does not want her family to come and visit her. Mary's carers are worried because she does not try to eat anything and they see her getting very weak. Georgina, who trained in person-centred counselling, tries to help Mary.

a Explain some of the ways in which Georgina can try to get Mary to talk to her.

b Discuss the benefits of person-centred counselling for someone like Mary.

12.8 Choosing an approach

This important topic summarises the four approaches we have studied and highlights the differences between them. Each approach is evaluated in turn, with advantages and disadvantages discussed. It is important to realise that each approach has its place and that there are instances where more than one approach would be appropriate. It should be emphasised that each approach has its supporters and its critics.

The *Getting you thinking* questions are designed to help students see that there are many reasons why people might 'cry', and not all of these might be because they are unhappy. They also give the students an opportunity to say what they think about the use of each of the approaches. This should stimulate a robust discussion about the suitability of the different approaches depending on a client's age and circumstances.

Answers to the *Check your understanding* questions on page 287 of the Collins textbook.

1 **Clinical psychologists have a code of conduct which sets out standards of professional behaviour, to protect the rights and interests of the people they work with. A professional code of conduct is similar to a care value base: they both highlight the sort of behaviour that is expected from care professionals. A code of conduct is likely to be more detailed and formal.**

2 **Two advantages of a behavioural approach are: the basic idea is easy to understand, and it is objective – with everyone able to see the relevant behaviour. Disadvantages of a behavioural approach are: it ignores what is going on inside the person's head, and it only deals with the symptoms and not the causes of people's problems.**

3 **A 'false memory syndrome' in psychodynamic therapy is where people undergoing analysis claim to have recovered memories of traumatic and abusive episodes from their childhood that did not actually occur.**

4 **A cognitive-behaviour approach might be used in health and care settings where people have difficulty coping with life – with issues such as stress, depression, anxieties and anger management.**

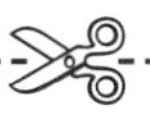

These questions guide you through the topic. If you need help to answer them, look at pages 282–287 of the Collins textbook.

12.8 short questions and activities

1 List the four major approaches that psychologists have used to understand human behaviour.

2 Which type of approach is usually used with a very young client? Why do you think this is the case?

3 What is meant by 'fuzzy' words, and why would these not be used in a behavioural approach?

4 What is significant about the fact that the behavioural approach assumes that nearly all of our behaviour is learnt?

5 Give one advantage and one disadvantage of a psychodynamic approach.

6 Give one similarity between a cognitive (cognitive-behavioural) approach and a behavioural approach.

7 Give one similarity between a cognitive (cognitive-behavioural) approach and a psychodynamic approach.

8 Give one similarity between a humanistic (person-centred) approach and a cognitive (cognitive-behavioural) approach.

9 Explain which two types of approach may be described as 'deterministic'.

summary worksheet

SORTING OUT THE APPROACHES

Here is a list of the four main approaches, along with an associated technique for dealing with problematic behaviour.

• **Behavioural**	• behaviour modification
• **Cognitive**	• cognitive-behaviour therapy
• **Psychodynamic**	• psychoanalysis
• **Humanistic**	• person-centred counselling

a Name the approach to which each of the following descriptions applies:

i It uses positive reinforcement.

....

ii It has an emphasis on the 'unconscious mind'.

....

iii It is a 'talking therapy' where counsellors are not intrusive.

....

b Which two approaches pay particular attention to what a client says?

1 ....

2 ....

c Some approaches are likely to involve a longer period of therapy than others.

i Explain which approach is likely to involve the longest period of therapy.

....

....

....

ii Explain which approach is likely to involve the shortest period of therapy.

....

....

....

12.8 extension**activity**sheet

WHICH APPROACH TO USE?

This diagram shows some issues for a care professional to consider when working with a client.

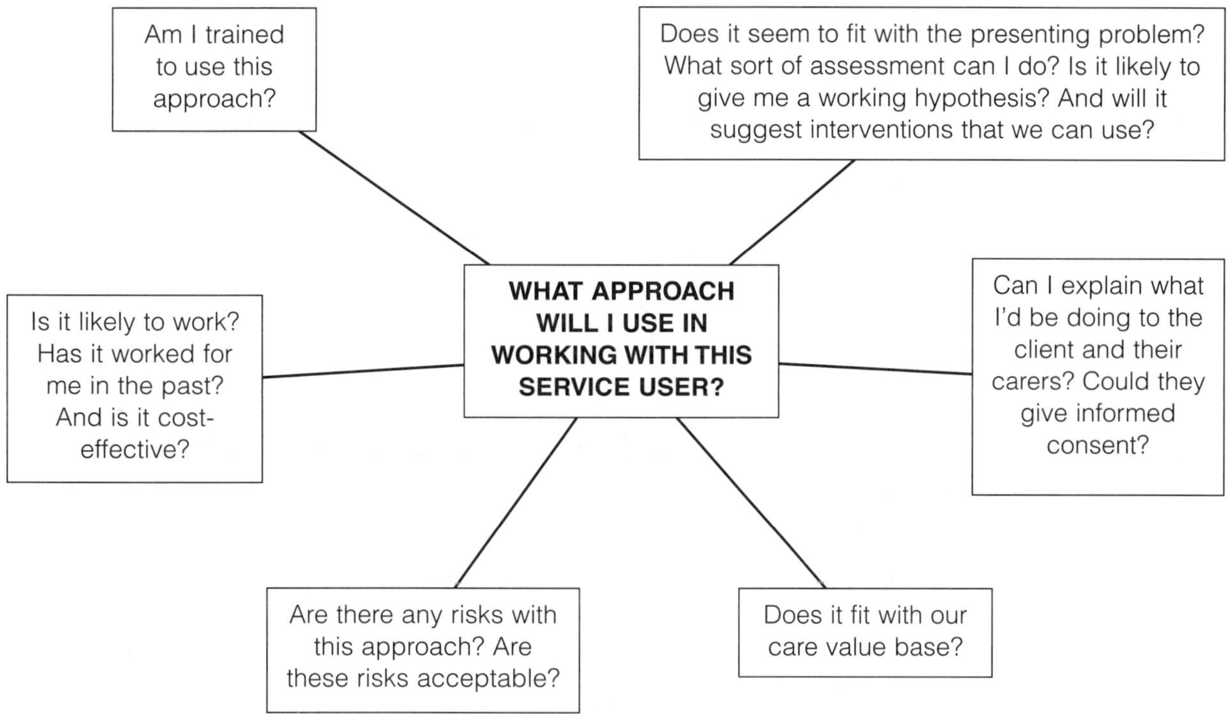

a Look at the six boxes and put them in order of importance, explaining your reasoning. You may find this task difficult – remember there are no correct answers.

b Make up a table that shows some advantages and disadvantages of each type of approach, along with examples of when the use of each approach would be particularly appropriate.

c Compare your answers to parts **a** and **b** with someone else in the class, and discuss reasons for any differences in your answers.

12.9 Seeing the approaches in practice

This topic is based on several case studies, each using a different psychological approach. Throughout the case studies, key words and concepts are emphasised. This should reinforce them for the student and show how the different approaches work in practice. The reasons for using a particular approach are explained and the students are encouraged to think of the advantages for the choice of approach used.

One of the case studies is introduced in the *Getting you thinking* section. The questions should prompt students to voice their opinions, based on what they have already learned. After studying the topic it would be useful to revisit these questions to see if the students' views have changed.

Answers to the *Check your understanding* questions on page 293 of the Collins textbook.

The answers to these have already been covered in earlier topics.

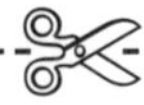

These questions guide you through the topic. If you need help to answer them, look at pages 288–293 of the Collins textbook.

12.9 short **questions** and **activities**

1. Identify Robbie's problem behaviour. Be as specific as you can.
2. Explain how the playgroup staff will positively reinforce Robbie's behaviour.
3. Give two practical reasons why Ken chooses cognitive (cognitive-behavioural) therapy when working with Ann.
4. How do the four approaches deal with assessment?
5. What is meant by 'family therapy'? Explain when it is particularly useful.
6. What is a 'multi-agency meeting' in a health and social care setting? Explain the importance of such meetings.
7. Why does Dr McNeil think it is appropriate for Kate Buchanan, the social worker, to talk about Joan's behaviour when the meeting is discussing the care of Mrs O'Brien?

12.9 **summary**worksheet

CANDICE WANTS TO GIVE UP SMOKING – A CASE STUDY

Read the following case study and answer the questions that follow.

> Candice is 16 and has made a New Year resolution to give up smoking. She says she started smoking because it made her feel more grown-up – and most of her friends smoked. She has difficulty finding the money to buy cigarettes and recently got into trouble for stealing money from someone at school. Candice has low self-esteen and thinks that no one will want to be friends with her now. She knows that giving up smoking will be hard, but she is determined to do it. She has asked her mum, Sarah, who does not smoke, to help her.

a Explain why Candice started to smoke.

....

....

....

b Explain what is meant by low self-esteem.

....

....

....

c Explain the evidence that shows Candice has an internal locus of control.

....

....

....

d Discuss the different way that Sarah could help Candice to give up smoking.

....

....

....

....

....

....

extension**activity**sheet

WHAT TYPE OF APPROACH FOR AGATHA?

Read the following case study and answer the questions that follow.

> Agatha is 86 years of age. She lives in sheltered accommodation and uses a wheelchair. She believes that Marjorie, one of the other residents, does not like her because she ignores her when she tries to speak to her. She believes that Marjorie is turning all the other residents against her. Marjorie is deaf. She has always kept herself to herself and never seems to smile much. Agatha has started not going to the residents' lounge and spends most of her time in her room. She is lonely, but is afraid to go out. Marilyn, the manager of the residental home, wonders what she can do to help Agatha.

a Explain the evidence that some of Agatha's thinking is distorted.

b Explain why it is unlikely that a behavioural approach will work with Agatha.

c Give the advantages and disadvantages of using a psychoanalytical approach with Agatha.

d Discuss whether a cognitive (cognitive-behavioural) approach or a humanistic (person-centred) approach would be more appropriate for Agatha.

Glossary of Health & Social Care terms

ABC Approach (Behavioural) – This is a strategy for analysing behaviour. It involves looking at the Antecedents, Behaviour and Consequences of specific behaviours.

ABC Approach (Cognitive) – This is a strategy for analysing the links between thinking and behaviour. It involves analysing behaviour in terms of the Activating event, Beliefs (which may be irrational or dysfunctional) and the emotional or behavioural Consequences.

Absolute poverty – A level of income below that which will sustain good health.

Accountability – Being responsible to someone or for something. Registered health and social care practitioners are accountable, for example, to their professional body, as well as their employers, for the quality of their care practice.

Aetiology – The study of what causes a disease.

Age discrimination – Treating people differently (and normally less well) on the basis of their age.

Ageism – Attitudes and behaviour which discriminate against older people.

Aim – A person or an organisation's focus or intention. It refers to what they intend to achieve.

Alzheimer's disease – A form of dementia that leads to progressive degeneration of the brain and is the commonest cause of dementia in people of all ages.

Assessment – In health and social care, the assessment process typically involves identifying and judging a person's care needs or personal skills and abilities. In a broader sense the term can refer to the process of judging the importance or effectiveness of something (such as assessing a drug treatment or a health promotion activity).

Atheroma – Fatty plaques that form inside the lining of arteries.

Audit – The monitoring of current activity, practice or policy against predefined standards.

Bacterium – A single-celled micro-organism, capable of reproducing on its own.

Behavioural approach – This approach says that most of our behaviour is learned; it can be unlearned and re-learned using reinforcement (rewards).

Behaviour change – A change in the way someone acts or functions.

Behaviour modification programme – This involves using behavioural approaches to change someone's behaviour.

Beneficence – Acts of charity or generosity that go beyond what people are normally expected to do.

Benign tumour – A discrete lump of cells that is harmless.

Bereavement – Suffering loss as a result of someone dying.

Birth rate – The number of live births per thousand of the population in one year.

Bullying – Deliberate and repeated attempts to hurt or upset another person.

Care planning cycle/process – A multi-stage cycle used by care practitioners to produce and implement individualised care plans.

Care value base – The values and ethical principles that care practitioners apply to their work. These are based on beliefs about the proper way to treat service users. Confidentiality, respecting a person's beliefs and behaving in a non-discriminatory way are all examples of care values.

CAT scan – This refers to Computed Axial Tomography which is a diagnostic technique that involves taking X-rays linked up to a computer.

Census – A national headcount of people and households carried out within a given population.

Central government – The national, as opposed to the local, level of government.

Charters – Documents that set out the targets and standards of service that a care organisation seeks to achieve in its work with service users.

Client centred – This involves focusing on the individual needs, wishes and preferences of clients to maximise their involvement in and control over their care.

Clinical features – The signs and symptoms of a disease.

Clinical governance – The process of improving the quality of care services by controlling and improving work systems in a care organisation.

Clinical trial – An experiment that tries out a potentially helpful procedure on human volunteers in order to find out how well the procedure may or may not work. A clinical trial also attempts to discover and assess risks that may occur during and/or after the procedure.

Cognitive – This term refers to thoughts and thinking.

Cognitive-behavioural therapy (CBT) – A form of treatment that uses a cognitive approach to help people change the way they feel and act.

Cognitive development – The development of thinking and understanding skills.

Cognitive primacy – The view that what we think determines what we feel and do.

Commission for Social Care Inspection (CSCI) – This body monitors, inspects and regulates standards of care in the social care sector in England.

Commissioning – The acquisition or purchasing of care services on behalf of a local population of people.

Communicable disease – A disease caused by a micro-organism which can be transmitted from one person to another.

Community Care – Provision where people should be cared for in their homes or in small 'family' units rather than in large, less personal institutions.

Comparative need – A person's needs in comparison with others in the same situation.

Complementary and alternative medicine – This term is used to describe a diverse range of health-focused practices and treatments, including acupuncture, reflexology and herbal medicine, that are not currently part of orthodox or conventional medicine.

Compliance – The extent to which a patient follows the medical or health advice that they have been given.

Concordance – This term is used to refer to agreement between patient and doctor.

Congruence – This refers to a matching or 'fit' between our experiences and our expectations or self-concept.

Conscious – What we are aware of.

Consultant – A highly skilled, expert care worker who specialises in a particular condition, disease or area of practice.

Control group – A group that is not exposed to a new drug or intervention during a clinical trial but which is compared to a group that is.

Convenience sample – A sample of individuals that is selected for reasons of convenience. That is, the individuals are chosen because they fit the researcher's selection criteria but are not chosen randomly.

Core conditions for person-centred therapy – This refers to the relationship that the counsellor tries to create, based on unconditional positive regard, empathy and genuineness.

Coronary arteries – Blood vessels supplying the heart muscle with food and oxygen.

Counselling – This refers to the supportive process of helping someone (a client) to analyse personal experiences, relationships or issues that are affecting their feelings or their behaviour.

Culture of poverty – A view that poverty is associated with a particular, and separate way of life that is passed on from generation to generation.

Data – Facts that might consist of observations, measurements or other factual information.

Data analysis – The procedures that scientists use to make sense of the data that they collect.

Death rate – The number of deaths per thousand of the population in one year.

Dementia – A group of diseases where there is a progressive loss of brain function.

Demography – The systematic study of the growth, size, distribution, movement and composition of human populations.

Dependent population – The age groups who are dependent on the rest of the population for economic security, namely young people from 0–16 years and those over the retirement age.

Dependency culture – The view that a welfare state will create a society where people rely on state benefits and services rather than working, planning for the future and taking responsibility for their own lives.

Descriptive statistics – Statistics that enable researchers to describe *what* the data are, without drawing conclusions about why this is so.

Deterministic theories – These are theories that see our behaviour as being caused (determined) by things we have no control over. These kind of theories would say that we have no free-will – that is, we think we make choices, but we don't.

Devolved system – Devolution occurs where central government grants power to government at regional or local level. A devolved system is one based on the devolution of power.

DHSSPS – This is an acronym for the Department of Health, Social Services and Public Safety, which has overall responsibility for health and care policy in Northern Ireland.

Diagnosis – The way that practitioners identify and classify a disorder or a disease.

Direct payments – The arrangement whereby a cash payment is made to people who have been assessed as needing community care services. They are then able to select, and pay for, the specific support they need, using the direct payment.

Disabling environment – A physical environment or social situation that presents barriers to access or which prevents participation by certain people.

Discrimination – Treating a person or a group of people differently and usually less favourably than others.

Distributive justice – This refers to the fair distribution of goods and services according to need.

Double-blind assignment – Assignment of people to experimental and control groups such that neither the researcher nor the participants know who is in which group while the research study is being carried out.

DSM-IV – The fourth revision of the Diagnostic and Statistical Manual of the American Psychiatric Association. It has nearly 300 categories of mental disorders.

Dysfunctional beliefs – Beliefs which are thought to be faulty and unhelpful to the person who holds them.

Egalitarian society – A society in which everyone is regarded as equal.

Ego – A term used in psychodynamic approaches that refers to the part of our mind that is rational and based in reality.

Ego defence mechanisms – The ways the ego can protect itself from the urges of the id (the part of our mind that contains our basic instincts, aggressive and sexual drives) – repression, for example.

Eligibility criteria – The requirements or standards that must be met before a person is provided with a care service.

Emigration – This refers to people leaving this country to live in another country.

Empathy – The ability to see and feel things from another person's point of view.

Empirical evidence – Evidence based on direct observation and experience.

Empowerment – A process of supporting and giving choice and decision-making powers to individuals or groups.

Endoscope – A fibre-optic tube for seeing inside the body. This is often used, for example, to examine the state of a person's digestive tract.

Epidemiology – The study of the spread of disease and causes of death and disability in a population.

Ethics – A code of behaviour based on moral principles.

Evaluation – This is the process of finding or judging the value or significance of something. For example, care practitioners evaluate the effectiveness of the interventions and treatments that they use.

Evidence-based practice – Practice that applies the best available evidence, some of it available from research studies, some of it gained from practical experience.

Expectation of life – A statistical measure which predicts the average number of years a person is likely to live. This is often calculated from birth but could be estimated from a particular age.

Experiment – A research procedure that exposes one of two samples to an intervention (e.g. a new medical treatment) in order to see if the intervention has an effect.

Experimental group – A group that is exposed to an intervention.

Exploratory question – A question that encourages an open investigation of a subject or issue.

Expressed need – The needs that people themselves identify and ask for assistance with.

Extended family – This term refers to a family or group, of normally three or more generations, who form a close-knit network and provide support and care for members.

External locus of control – The belief that we have little control over events; where control is believed to be external to, outside of, us. People who believe their future will be decided by 'fate', chance or an 'act of God' rather than by their own actions are likely to have an external locus of control.

Extinguishing behaviour – This refers to eliminating unwanted behaviour through specific steps.

Felt need – What people feel they need.

Functional beliefs – These are ways of thinking that are helpful to us.

Fungus – Usually a multi-cellular micro-organism with a thread-like structure, e.g. mould, but sometimes exists as a single cell, e.g. yeast.

Genuineness – Giving something of yourself in a therapeutic relationship so that there is congruence between what you say, how you present yourself and what you do, think and feel.

Governance of research – The process of applying and monitoring approved research 'rules' and procedures.

GP fund-holding – A funding system where general practitioners are given a budget to spend on purchasing care for patients on their practice list.

Hawthorne effect – This refers to the tendency of participants to behave differently when they know they are being studied.

Health and Social Services Boards – These are the main purchasing or commissioning bodies in Northern Ireland.

Health and Social Services Trusts – These are the main providers of statutory care services in Northern Ireland.

Healthcare Commission – This body monitors, inspects and regulates standards of care in the health care sector.

Holistic assessment – An assessment that focuses on the 'whole person' rather than a specific or partial aspect of their functioning.

Homework – The tasks the client is asked to do – things to practise until they see the counsellor again.

Hypertensive – Having persistent high blood pressure.

Hypotheses – Intelligent but untested propositions.

ICD – International Classification of Diseases.

Id – The part of our mind that contains our basic instincts, and our aggressive and sexual drives (according to psychodynamic approaches).

Immigration – This refers to people coming to live in this country from another country.

Impairment – The limitations that may be made on an individual due to physical, mental or sensory dysfunction.

Incidence – The number of new cases of a specified disease occurring in a given period of time.

Inclusive design (or **Universal design**) – The design of products and environments for use by all people, to the greatest possible extent, without the need for adaptation or specialised design.

Independent living – A philosophy which holds that people with disabilities have the right to live with dignity and with appropriate support in their own homes, to participate fully in their communities, and to have control over their lives.

Independent sector – This term refers to private and not-for-profit voluntary care organisations that are independent of government. A collective term for the private and the voluntary care sectors.

Individualised care – Care that is planned and delivered to meet the specific needs of an individual.

Industrialisation – The development of an economy based on the production of goods in factories, mills and mines rather than agriculture and other cottage industries.

Infant mortality rate – The number of deaths of infants under 1 year of age per thousand live births.

Inferential statistics – Statistics that enable researchers to make inferences from their data to more general conditions.

Informal care – This is care that is provided by relatives and friends of the person who has care needs, on an unpaid basis, outside of the professional care system.

Informal carer – Someone who provides informal care.

Insecure attachment – A situation where someone fails to establish an effective emotional bond or close relationship, usually as a result of parental separation or the death of a parent or loved one.

Instinct – This term refers to those 'inbuilt' or innate ways of behaving and responding that we are born with.

Institutionalisation – This refers to the process of becoming dependent on the rules and routines of large organisations.

Internal locus of control – The belief that we are able to influence and even control events and outcomes in our lives.

Internal market – This is a 'market' in care services that was introduced to promote competition between statutory and other care providers in the early 1990s.

Inter-professional working – This term describes team-working arrangements where care practitioners with different disciplinary backgrounds work collaboratively to meet and manage the care needs of a service user or client.

Interventions – These are the strategies we use to try to resolve a problem or to provide care.

Interview guide – A basic checklist of themes that guides an interviewer on the particular issues that they should explore.

Labelling – The process of attaching stigmatising stereotypes to particular groups of people who are then seen as all sharing negative characteristics.

Laissez-faire – This is a view that the government should not interfere in the workings of the economy nor in the provision of welfare services. The government should 'leave well alone'.

Legislation – A collective term for laws that are passed by Parliament or the EU.

Life expectancy – The average number of years a person is likely to live from a particular point in time. Life expectancy is normally calculated from birth.

Local government – The local, as opposed to national, level of government.

Local Health Care Co-operatives – The bodies that have responsibility for primary care in Scotland.

Locus – The Latin word for 'place'.

Malignant tumour – Lumps of cells that can travel around the body and grow in various organs, also referred to as cancer.

Mass media – This refers to forms of communication, such as television, radio and national newspapers, that are designed to reach a large or mass audience.

Matching – A procedure that helps to ensure that any 'extreme' characteristic in an experimental group (someone with an eating disorder, for example) has a match (counterpart) in the control group.

Means tested benefits – Welfare benefits which are only available to people if their income and savings are below a level decided by government.

Medication – Tablets or other forms of prescribed drugs given to aid recovery.

Meta-analysis – A quantitative systematic review.

Mission statement – A formal statement of a care organisation's aims or objectives. It sets out the organisation's sense of purpose or 'mission'.

Mixed economy of care – A care system that combines public (government), private, voluntary and informal sector services. Each of these types of care is funded in a different way, hence the term 'mixed economy'.

Monoclonal antibodies – 'Magic bullets' designed to 'fight' disease-causing organisms within the body.

Morality – This refers to moral ideas about 'goodness' and 'badness'.

Morbidity – This refers to experiences of ill-health.

Morbidity rate – The number of people who have a particular illness or disease in a given population and at a particular time.

Mortality rate – The number of people who have died from a particular disease in a given population and time.

MRI scan – Magnetic Resonance Imaging, a diagnostic technique using magnetism that produces clear scans.

Multi-agency working – A situation where care practitioners employed by different care organisations (or 'agencies') collaborate to provide care for a particular individual or group of people.

Multi-disciplinary team – A team of care workers from a range of professional backgrounds. This may include doctors, nurses, social workers and occupational therapists, for example.

Multiple Sclerosis – A condition where the immune system attacks and destroys the nerves resulting in the gradual, and eventually terminal, loss of physical functioning.

Myelin sheath – The insulating material that surrounds the nerves.

National Service Frameworks – These are service standards for specific areas of care practice that are defined by government. Care organisations are expected to provide and achieve levels of service delivery that meet these standards.

Need – Something a person requires or could benefit from. People have physical, intellectual, emotional and social needs.

Negative reinforcement – The removal of an aversive or unpleasant stimulus.

Net migration – The difference between the number of immigrants and the number of emigrants.

New Right, The – A view that the government should play a minimal role in the provision of welfare. Taxes should be low and people should decide how they spend their money, making their own provision for health and welfare needs.

Non-communicable disease – A disease not caused by a micro-organism and not usually passed from one person to another.

Non-invasive technique – A diagnostic or treatment procedure that does not involve piercing, cutting or entering the body.

Normative need – Established or expected levels or definitions of 'need', typically defined by academic 'experts' or professional practitioners.

Northern Ireland Assembly – The body (currently suspended) that is due to take on central government responsibilities in Northern Ireland.

Nuclear family – The smaller family unit of two generations – parent(s) and their children.

Nuclear imaging – Using a gamma camera and radionuclides to view abnormal function in the body, e.g. cancer cells.

Objective – This is a specific, clearly identified target to achieve.

Observation – In qualitative research, this procedure usually refers to watching people in their natural settings.

Open-ended interview – An informal interview in which the sequence and wording of the questions are not decided in advance.

Ophthalmic – Relating to the eye.

Organisational culture – The values, beliefs and assumptions that influence the practices and procedures or ways of working and 'atmosphere' of an organisation.

Organismic self – A version of the self that contains everything we experience, including things we are not aware of.

Osteoarthritis – A degenerative disease affecting the cartilage of the joints, often occurring after injury.

Paramountcy principle – The principle of putting the welfare of the child first in all decisions affecting them.

Parkinson's disease – A slowly progressing disease of the nervous system that results in involuntary tremors and the loss of muscular control and movement abilities.

Pathology – The scientific study of disease, but also a term used to describe something that is abnormal.

PET scan – Positron Emission Tomography, a diagnostic technique similar to a CAT scan, useful for diagnosing brain tumours, but expensive.

Philanthropy – The practice of helping people who are less well-off than oneself. It is associated with the charitable work of very wealthy people and played an important part in the emergence of voluntary organisations in the Victorian era.

Placebo – An inactive substance or procedure that resembles the experimental intervention being studied.

Placebo effect – The tendency of some participants to think they have been affected by a research intervention even though they haven't been. This occurs because they know about the aim of the research in which they are involved and are suggestible.

Population – The total of all persons who possess a common characteristic that is being studied (e.g. all poor children in Birmingham).

Positive reinforcement – This is any form of pleasant stimulus that has the effect of increasing the likely recurrence of a particular behaviour.

Post-industrial society – An economy based less on the manual production of goods but rather on non-manual work through the service, and office-based, occupations.

Poverty line – A term introduced by Seebohm Rowntree which set a level of income, below which people were said to be in poverty.

Prejudice – A strongly held attitude towards a particular group which will often persist even when shown to be unjustified or unfounded.

Prescription – In medical practice this refers to written instructions from a qualified doctor for the making-up and use of a medicine or treatment.

Pressure group – interest group organised to influence public, and especially government, policy.

Prevalence – The total number of cases of a specified disease occurring in a population at a particular point in time.

Primary care – This is 'first line' or 'first contact' care, usually provided by community-based health care workers such as general practitioners (GPs) or District Nurses. Typically, primary care involves the diagnosis of health symptoms, the treatment of 'everyday' and less serious complaints and referral of more complex cases to secondary care providers.

Primary Care Trust – Public sector organisations that monitor and manage the work of primary care providers in a local area.

Primary Health Care – Care provided by a care worker such as a GP, usually the first person to help a client.

Primary research – Research that produces new or 'fresh' data.

Private care/sector – Care services that are provided to people who are willing and able to pay for them. Organisations and individual practitioners who sell care services in this way are known as the 'private sector'.

Private practitioners – Care practitioners who are either self-employed or who are employed by a private sector care organisation.

Professional referral – A request by one care professional for care services to be provided by another care professional.

Provider organisation – A care organisation that delivers care services directly to service users.

Psychiatrist – A medical doctor who has specialist training and qualifications that allow them to work with people experiencing mental distress.

Psychodynamic approaches – Approaches that believe that our thoughts and feelings are the result of unconscious processes.

Psychology – The systematic study of how people think, feel and behave.

Punishment – This refers to the deliberate use or application of an unpleasant stimulus.

Purchaser organisation – An organisation that commissions or buys care services on behalf of an individual or group of people.

Qualitative – This term is used for methods of assessment that describe the outcomes in words rather than numbers.

Qualitative data – Non-numerical data, usually presented as 'talk' or 'text', though it can also include images and objects which provide some form of information or evidence.

Quality assurance – A general process of monitoring and evaluating whether specified standards of service quality have been achieved.

Quality standards – Statements of performance or outcomes that define an acceptable level of service.

Quantitative – The term used for methods of assessment that are numerical.

Quantitative data – Information presented in numerical form. Typically this involves some form of quantifiable measure.

Quasi-experiment – A research study that is based on, or mimics, the experimental method but which doesn't fulfil all of the criteria required in closely controlled experimental research.

Radionuclide – Low-level dose of a radioactive material.

Random sample – A sample of individuals selected from a population where all have an equal chance of being chosen.

Regulatory – This refers to monitoring and control.

Reinforcement – This refers to something (like a reward) that follows something we've done, which makes that behaviour more likely to happen again.

Relative poverty – Relative poverty occurs when people live below the standard of living normally accepted in a particular society.

Reliable results – Findings that can be confirmed by other scientists.

Research-based evidence – Findings that are based on data collected through systematic investigation.

Review – This refers to the process of checking to see how well an intervention has worked.

Rheumatism – A musculo-skeletal condition that causes pain in a person's muscles and joints and which can lead to deformity of the joints.

Rheumatoid arthritis – A degenerative disease affecting the joints where the body's immune system attacks itself.

Rogerian counselling – Person-centred counselling, in the style of Carl Rogers.

Role – The job, task or function that a person has.

Sample – A portion of some people in a population.

Schedule of reinforcement – This refers to how often a specific behaviour is reinforced.

Schemas – This refers to how we bring together and organise information about ourselves and things around us.

Schematic thinking – Thinking using schemas.

Science – A way of knowing, based upon testing the truthfulness of ideas against empirical evidence.

Scottish Parliament – The body that has central government responsibilities in Scotland.

Secondary care – Health care services that are provided by hospital-based specialists for people with more complex or emergency health care needs.

Secondary data – Existing data that has been collected and analysed by a previous researcher but which can be reanalysed and reused in a subsequent research study.

Secondary research – Typically, research based on the analysis of existing, secondary data or which focuses on finding this kind of data.

Secure attachment – This is where the young child feels safe and secure with their preferred carer.

Self-actualisation – The process of becoming a whole, complete person.

Self-referral – A direct request by an individual for health care services. Going to see a GP is an example of a self-referral.

Shaping behaviour – Building up complex patterns of behaviour gradually, in small steps.

Signs – Characteristics of a disease detectable by another person.

Social class –There are many competing definitions of social class. Central to all definitions is the idea that a person's position in society is determined by their economic circumstances that will then influence their life choices, opportunities and future prospects.

Social exclusion – A term used to describe a situation where people are unable to participate fully in society for a number of related reasons, often including poverty, unemployment, poor housing or homelessness, poor health and poor educational achievement.

Socialisation – This is the process of learning how our society works, its expectations and rules.

Social reinforcement – Any form of praise, attention and recognition that we get from others which encourages us to repeat desired behaviour.

Social stratification – The grouping of people together according to their perceived status or rank within the society.

Societal change – This refers to changes in the structure and processes of a society.

Sociology – The study of social structures and processes.

Statute – An Act of Parliament.

Statutory care/sector – Care services that have to be provided by law. They are usually provided by public or government-controlled care organisations such as NHS trusts.

Stereotype – Defining a group of people, e.g. black people or lone parents, as if they all possess the same personal characteristics, ignoring their individual differences.

Stigma – Negative attitudes which lead to the unfavourable treatment of particular groups.

Superego – The part of our mind that represents ideals and values; our conscience.

Survey – A method for obtaining information from a sample of a population.

Symptoms – Characteristics of a disease felt by the person that have no physical manifestation.

Symptom substitution – This happens when one behaviour (e.g. nail-biting) is extinguished, only to be replaced by another (e.g. bed-wetting).

Synthesised – Combined or brought together into a detailed summary.

Systematic review – A systematic analysis of other analyses.

Task-focused care – Forms of care that focus on carrying out a series of specified tasks for one or more service users, such as 'toileting everyone at 3 p.m.', regardless of the service users' individual care needs.

Team-building – The process of developing a group of employees into an effective work team.

Theory – The set of linked and abstract ideas we use to understand and explain things. Some theories allow us to predict and control events.

Third Way, The – An approach to welfare that tries to combine individual freedom and responsibility with a state providing for those most in need.

Time out – This is strategy for dealing with inappropriate behaviour that involves removing someone from all sources of social reinforcement until their inappropriate behaviour ends.

Transmission of disease – The passing of a disease from one person to another.

Token economy – Using tokens (stars, smiley faces) as reinforcement. The tokens have no value in themselves, but can be exchanged for something the person wants.

Total institutions – A large, highly organised residential establishment where people live their lives separate from the wider society, e.g. prison or army barracks or large psychiatric hospital.

Total Quality Management – A management philosophy that seeks to integrate all of the functions of an organisation (marketing, finance, care delivery, customer service, etc.) in a way that focuses on meeting customer needs and the organisation's objectives.

Transactional analysis (TA) – An approach to understanding behaviour through interpreting the interactions people have.

Typology – This is a classification system that identifies 'types' of something.

Ultrasound – A diagnostic technique that uses high-frequency sound to view soft tissues inside the body.

Unconditional positive regard – Acceptance and respect; being non-judgemental.

Unconscious – Thoughts and feelings that we are not aware of.

Underclass – A term coined by Gunnar Myrdal (1969) closely linked with the idea of social exclusion, normally used now to refer to the people in poverty who are excluded from fully participating in society by social and economic changes which are outside their control.

Unfair discrimination – The unjustified and less favourable treatment of a person or a group, perhaps as a result of prejudice.

Universal benefits – Welfare benefits to which people are entitled, regardless of their income or savings.

Urban living – A society where a high proportion of the population live and work in towns and cities rather than living and working off the land in agricultural communities.

Valid results – Findings that are based on the most appropriate research instruments.

Vector – An organism that transfers disease-causing micro-organisms from one person to another, e.g. mosquito or rat.

Vicarious reinforcement – Indirect reinforcement.

Victim blaming – Being held responsible for one's own misfortune.

Virus – Very small micro-organism with a simple structure.

Voluntary care/sector – Care services that are provided free of charge or for a small, subsidised fee by non-profit making organisations.

Welfare state – A term, first used during the 1940s, to refer to a system in which government took a primary responsibility for the health and welfare of the nation through the provision or monitoring of services.

Working hypothesis – An attempt to understand what is causing or contributing to a problem.

